GW00658261

Get Through

New MRCGP: Applied Knowledge Test

Una Coales

MD FRCS FRCS(ENT) DRCOG DFFP MRCGP
Sole Educator/Course Organiser of
www.mrcgpcourses.co.uk
Primary Access Support GP for the Lambeth PCT
Executive Committee Member of the South London Faculty of
the Royal College of General Practitioners

The ROYAL
SOCIETY *of*
MEDICINE
PRESS *Limited*

© 2007 Royal Society of Medicine Press Ltd

Published by the Royal Society of Medicine Press Ltd
1 Wimpole Street, London W1G 0AE, UK
Tel: +44 (0)20 7290 2921
Fax: +44 (0)20 7290 2929
Email: publishing@rsm.ac.uk
Website: www.rsmpress.co.uk

Apart from any fair dealing for the purposes of research or private study, criticism or review, as permitted under the UK Copyright, Designs and Patents Act, 1988, no part of this publication may be reproduced, stored or transmitted, in any form or by any means, without the prior permission in writing of the publishers or in the case of reprographic reproduction in accordance with the terms of licences issued by the Copyright Licensing Agency in the UK, or in accordance with the terms of licences issued by the appropriate Reproduction Rights Organization outside the UK. Enquiries concerning reproduction outside the terms stated here should be sent to the publishers at the UK address printed on this page.

The right of Una Coales to be identified as author of this work has been asserted by her in accordance with the Copyright, Designs and Patents Act, 1988.

British Library Cataloguing in Publication Data
A catalogue record for this book is available from the British Library

ISBN 978-1-85315-775-2

Distribution in Europe and Rest of World:
Marston Book Services Ltd
PO Box 269
Abingdon
Oxon OX14 4YN, UK
Tel: +44 (0)1235 465500
Fax: +44 (0)1235 465555
Email: direct.order@marston.co.uk

Distribution in the USA and Canada:
Royal Society of Medicine Press Ltd
c/o BookMasters Inc
30 Amberwood Parkway
Ashland, OH 44805, USA
Tel: +1 800 247 6553/+1 800 266 5564
Fax: +1 419 281 6883
Email: orders@bookmasters.com

Distribution in Australia and New Zealand:
Elsevier Australia
30-52 Smidmore Street
Marrikville NSW 2204, Australia
Tel: +61 2 9517 8999
Fax: +61 2 9517 2249
Email: service@elsevier.com.au

Typeset by Phoenix Photosetting, Chatham, Kent
Printed and bound in Great Britain by Bell & Bain Ltd, Glasgow

Contents

Preface

As of August 2007, GPs will be required to obtain the new MRCGP (nMRCGP, as it will be known during the phasing-in period) by the end of their third year of specialist training to be licensed as a GP and receive a certificate of completion of training (CCT). The new MRCGP consists of three components:

1. an applied knowledge test (AKT) – similar content and format as the current MCQ paper
2. a clinical skills assessment (CSA) – 14 OSCE stations with simulated patients
3. a workplace-based assessment (WPBA).

GP trainees in specialist training have three attempts to pass this new exam. This replaces the old MRCGP exam, which will end in May 2008. Established GPs will be limited to obtaining membership through assessment of performance or MAP.

The AKT is modelled on the old MRCGP MCQ module (algorithms, extended matching questions, multiple best answers, single best answer, etc.), and candidates who have passed the old MCQ module may be eligible for credit towards the new MRCGP.

On this premise, I have put together questions based on the old MRCGP MCQ module and added new questions for your revision. Please use this book as an aide mémoire, i.e. if you read questions on Fitness to Drive, this should prompt you to read the Fitness to Drive guidance on www.dvla.gov.uk website. These are not identical questions to the actual exam but rather, they are very similar in topic content and format. The sources of the AKT questions will include the *Oxford Handbook* Series (*General Practice, Clinical Medicine, Clinical Specialties*), Office of National Statistics, NICE guidelines, BMJ Clinical Evidence and the *British National Formulary*.

Good luck!

Dr Una Coales
Sole Educator/Course Organiser of www.mrcgpcourses.co.uk
Primary Access Support GP for the Lambeth PCT
Executive Committee Member of the South London Faculty of the
Royal College of General Practitioners

Recommended texts and references

Coales U (2003). *Get Through MRCGP: New MCQ Module.* The Royal Society of Medicine Press Ltd., London.

Collier JAB, Longmore M, Brinsden M (2006). *Oxford Handbook of Clinical Specialties,* 7th edn. Oxford University Press, Oxford.

Davies T, Craig TKJ (1998). *ABC of Mental Health.* BMJ Books, London.

Department of Health (1999). *Drug Misuse and Dependence – Guidelines on Clinical Management.* HMSO, London.

DVLA (2006). *Fitness to Drive Guidelines.* (www.dvla.gov.uk)

Glasier A, Gebbie A. (2000). *Handbook of Family Planning and Reproductive Healthcare,* 4th edn. Churchill Livingstone, London.

Health and Safety Executive (2000). *Management of Health and Safety at Work Regulations 1999, Approved Code of Practice and Guidance.* HSE Books, London.

Longmore M, Wilkinson IB, Turmezei T, Cheung CK (2007). *Oxford Handbook of Clinical Medicine*, 7th edn. Oxford University Press, Oxford.

McLatchie GR, Leaper DJ (2002). *Oxford Handbook of Clinical Surgery*, 2nd edn. Oxford University Press, Oxford.

National Institute for Health and Clinical Excellence. NICE guidances. (www.nice.org.uk)

Neighbour R (2004). *The Inner Consultation*, 2nd edn. Radcliffe Publishing, Oxford.

Roland NJ, McRae RDR, McCombe AW. (2000). *Key Topics in Otolaryngology*, 2nd edn. BIOS Scientific Publishers, Oxford.

Royal Pharmaceutical Society of Great Britain (2007). *British National Formulary.* British Medical Association, London.

Simon C, Everitt H (2006) *Oxford Handbook of General Practice*, 2nd edn. Oxford University Press, Oxford.

Applied Knowledge Test Module Paper One: Questions

1. MBA. For which of the following conditions does the Department of Health recommend pneumococcal vaccination? (Source: *BNF*)

    A. Asplenia
    B. Cirrhosis
    C. Coeliac disease
    D. Diabetes mellitus
    E. Nephrotic syndrome

2. MBA. Viagra is licensed on the NHS and endorsed as 'SLS' to treat erectile dysfunction in men who have which of the following conditions? (Source: *BNF*):

    A. Diabetes mellitus
    B. Multiple sclerosis
    C. Parkinson's disease
    D. Prostate cancer
    E. Renal transplant

3–7. Anatomy of the tympanic membrane

    A. Incus
    B. Light reflex
    C. Manubrium of malleus
    D. Pars flaccida
    E. Pars tensa
    F. Stapedius
    G. Uncus

    Label the parts of the tympanic membrane shown below from the list above:

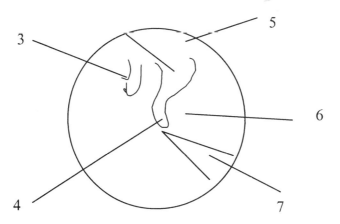

8–14. Match the following child development milestones:

A. 6 weeks
B. 12 weeks
C. 6 months
D. 7 months
E. 8 months
F. 9 months
G. 12 months
H. 18 months
I. 2 years
J. 3 years
K. 4 years
L. 5 years

8. Able to transfer cube from hand to hand.

9. Able to sit without support.

10. Able to hop on one foot.

11. Follows object 1 metre away.

12. Able to speak 10–12 words.

13. Knows first and last name.

14. Turns head to sounds level with the ear.

15–19. Fitness to drive (www.dvla.org.uk)

A. No driving licence restrictions
B. 1 month off driving
C. 6 months off driving
D. 12 months off driving
E. Permanently barred and requires DVLA notification
F. Refusal or revocation
G. Driving must cease until cause identified
H. Relicensing when symptom-free for 6/52

Match the following scenarios with the appropriate fitness-to-drive regulations:

15. A 22-year-old tour coach driver tests positive for HIV and has a CDC count.

16. A 40-year-old HGV driver presents with chest pain. He is referred for an exercise–stress test and is able to complete three stages of the Bruce protocol on exercise–stress test without anti-anginal medication and is free from signs of cardiovascular dysfunction.

17. A 40-year-old IVDA reports that he blacked out at the wheel and hit a tree. He has had no further episodes of syncope. He states that his tongue is sore.

18. A 55-year-old man has suffered a myocardial infarction. He has been treated and has undergone CABG.

19. A 60-year-old man suffers a stroke. He recovers.

20. Initial treatment recommendation for scabies is as follows: (*BNF*)
    A. Apply malathion 0.5% preparation over entire body after a hot bath and wash off after 12 hours. Repeat in 1 week's time.
    B. Apply benzoyl benzoate over the whole body; repeat without bathing on the following day and wash off 24 hours later. Repeat for up to 3 consecutive days.
    C. Apply permethrin 5% dermal cream over whole body and wash off after 12 hours. Repeat in 1 week's time.
    D. Prescribe ivermectin as a single dose of 200 µg/kg by mouth.
    E. Apply carbaryl lotion over whole body after hot bath and wash off after 24 hours. Repeat once a week for 3 consecutive weeks.

21–25. Sickness certificates (*Guidance Notes on Medical Certificates*)
    A. med 3
    B. med 4
    C. med 5
    D. med 6
    E. RM7
    F. DS 1500

21. This statement is completed if the doctor doubts the incapacity of the patient.

22. This statement of incapacity to work allows a return to work date to be given not more than 2 weeks after the date of the examination.

23. This statement is requested prior to a Personal Capacity Assessment.

24. This statement is for backdated medical certificates on the basis of a recent written report from another doctor.

25. This statement is issued for patients with terminal illness, who are likely to die within 6 months.

26–32. Match the following Sections of the Mental Health Act:

A. Section 2
B. Section 3
C. Section 4
D. Section 5
E. Section 7
F. Section 115
G. Section 135
H. Section 136

26. This gives police the right to remove a person from a public place to a place of safety, i.e. a prison cell or hospital for 72 hours to permit medical examination.

27. This gives a social worker the right of entry into a person's premises.

28. This allows one doctor to detain an inpatient for up to 72 hours in an emergency situation. A psychiatrist must then be contacted.

29. This permits compulsory emergency admission to hospital for 72 hours and requires one doctor who has seen the person in the last 24 hours plus a social worker or family member.

30. This requires 2 doctors (one of whom is section 12-approved) to admit a patient to hospital for up to 28 days for assessment and is not renewable.

31. This gives police the right of entry into premises to remove a person to a place of safety under a magistrate's warrant.

32. This requires 2 doctors (one of whom is section 12-approved) to admit a patient to hospital for up to 6 months for treatment and is renewable.

33–38. Algorithm for dyspepsia according to the British Society of Gastroenterology:

A. Age over 55 years presenting with new episode of dyspepsia and no alarm signs
B. Double-contrast barium meal (DCBM)
C. Endoscopic findings
D. Offer *Helicobacter pylori* serology
E. PPI
F. Refer to specialist
G. Return to self-care
H. Review
I. Significant acute GI bleed
J. Suspend NSAID use and review medication
K. Triple therapy for *H. pylori*
L. Urea breath test

Flowchart of referral criteria and subsequent management

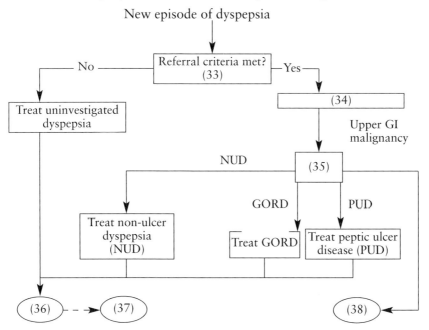

39. According to the NICE guideline on dyspepsia, urgent specialist referral for endoscopic investigation is indicated for patients of any age with dyspepsia when presenting with any of the following except:

   A. Chronic GI bleeding
   B. Epigastric mass
   C. Iron deficiency anaemia
   D. Persistent symptoms despite *H. pylori* testing and acid suppression therapy
   E. Persistent vomiting
   F. Progressive difficulty swallowing
   G. Progressive unintentional weight loss

40. According to the British Thoracic Society Guidelines for the management of stable COPD, the following treatment is advised for a 45-year-old man with breathlessness on exertion, cough and a 39% predicted FEV1:

   A. Regular combined inhaled short-acting β_2-agonists and anticholinergics and 30 mg oral prednisolone for 2 weeks
   B. Regular combined inhaled short-acting β_2-agonists and anticholinergics, corticosteroid trial and antibiotic therapy
   C. Regular inhaled short-acting β_2-agonists and regular inhaled anticholinergics, corticosteroid therapy and long-acting β_2-agonists
   D. Regular inhaled short-acting β_2-agonists or regular inhaled anticholinergics and consider corticosteroid therapy
   E. Theophylline and long-term oxygen therapy

41. Specialist referral in the management of COPD is required in the following situations:

   A. Bullous lung disease
   B. Cor pulmonale
   C. Family history of α_1-antitrypsin deficiency
   D. Oxygen therapy
   E. Uncertain diagnosis

42. Which evidence-based questionnaire is recommended for postnatal depression?

   A. Beck
   B. Edinburgh
   C. Hamilton
   D. Glasgow
   E. CAGE

43. Guidelines for urgent urology referral include:

   A. An elevated age-specific PSA in men with a 10-year life expectancy without signs of an active UTI
   B. Microscopic haematuria in adults over 50 years with irritative voiding symptoms
   C. Painful macroscopic haematuria in adults
   D. Palpable renal masses
   E. Swellings in the body of the testis

44. Guidelines for urgent referral to a colorectal clinic include:

   A. An easily palpable renal mass
   B. Change in bowel habits in a patient over 40 with previous polyps
   C. Iron deficiency anaemia with a normal upper endoscopy and a Hb of < 10g/dL
   D. Rectal bleeding and change in bowel habits in patients over 50 years of age
   E. Rectal bleeding and/or change in bowel habits in patients over 40 with ulcerative colitis

45. Cervical pap smear is recommended every 3 years for women between the ages of:

   A. 18–65
   B. 20–64
   C. 25–49
   D. 25–64
   E. 20–70

46. Breast cancer screening with mammography is recommended for women between the ages of:

   A. 40–60
   B. 45–60
   C. 45–65
   D. 50–60
   E. 50–64

47–51. Match the following ENT conditions:

   A. Acoustic neuroma
   B. Herpes zoster oticus
   C. Ménière's disease
   D. Occupational noise damage
   E. Otosclerosis
   F. Presbyacusis

47. A 35-year-old pregnant woman presents with bilateral conductive hearing loss. Both tympanic membranes appear normal.

48. A 70-year-old man presents with gradual onset of bilateral sensorineural hearing loss.

49. A 65-year-old woman presents with sudden onset of unilateral facial weakness and sensorineural hearing loss. She is also noted to have vesicles in the external auditory meatus.

50. A 50-year-old woman presents with unilateral low-frequency sensorineural hearing loss and vertigo.

51. A 50-year-old man presents with a gradual onset of unilateral sensorineural hearing loss and unilateral tinnitus.

52–56. Match the following drugs with the list of side effects: (Source: *BNF*)

    A. Altered colour vision
    B. Cataract
    C. Double vision
    D. Dry eyes
    E. Orange-red tears

52. Sildenafil

53. Propranolol

54. Carbamazepine

55. Prednisolone

56. Rifampicin

57–62. Match the following consultation models:

    A. Byrne and Long
    B. John Heron
    C. Roger Neighbour
    D. D. Pendleton
    E. M. Balint
    F. Eric Berne
    G. Stott and Davis

57. Connecting, summarizing, handing over, safety netting and house-keeping.

58. Management of present problems, modification of help-seeking behaviours, management of continuing problems and opportunistic health promotion.

59. Define the reason for the patient's attendance, consider other problems, choose an appropriate action with the patient, achieve a shared understanding, involve the patient in the management plan, use time and resources appropriately and establish a relationship with the patient that helps to achieve other tasks.

60. A study of 2500 audiotaped consultations identifying 'doctor-centred' and 'patient-centred' behaviours.

61. The spontaneous or dependent child, the logical adult, and the critical or caring parent.

62. The doctor as a drug, the child as the presenting complaint, elimination by appropriate physical examination, collusion of anonymity, the flash and the mutual investment company.

63. The Royal College of Physicians Guidelines for Oxygen Therapy recommends use of long-term oxygen therapy after specialist assessment for the following conditions:

A. COPD with $PaO_2 < 7.3$ kPa (on air)
B. Cystic fibrosis when $PaO_2 < 7.3$ kPa
C. Obstructive sleep apnoea despite continuous positive airways pressure therapy
D. Pulmonary hypertension without parenchymal lung involvement when $PaO_2 < 8$ kPa
E. Pulmonary malignancy with dyspnoea on moderate exertion

64. Contraindications to aromatherapy include which of the following (multiple best answer):

A. Contact dermatitis
B. Epilepsy
C. Exposure to the sun
D. First-trimester pregnancy
E. Hypertension
F. Homeopathy

65. Which **one** of the following statements regarding immunization is correct?

A. Anaphylactic reaction to egg ingestion contraindicates influenza and yellow fever vaccines.

B. Anaphylactic reaction to egg ingestion contraindicates MMR vaccine.

C. A personal or family history of inflammatory bowel disease contraindicates MMR vaccine.

D. Children given recent oral poliomyelitis vaccine should not be taken swimming.

E. Children given recent oral poliomyelitis vaccine contraindicates tonsillectomy.

66. Which **four** of the following statements regarding homeopathy are correct?

A. Belladonna is suggested for toothaches.

B. There are no contradictions to the use of homeopathy.

C. Homeopathy offers an alternative to the MMR vaccine.

D. Homeopathy was developed into a system of medicine by Dr Samuel Hahnemann in the late 18th century.

E. The principle of homeopathy uses the Law of Similars, i.e. when a substance used in large doses causes symptoms, in minute doses it can cure.

67–71. Match the following distribution graphs:

A. Bimodal

B. Equal means but different variances

C. Equal variances but different means

D. Negatively skewed

E. Normal

F. Positively skewed

67.

68.

69.

70.

71.

72. What is the **single** best initial drug treatment following a transient ischaemic attack?

A. Aspirin 75 mg od
B. Aspirin 75 mg od + dipyridamole 200 mg MR bd
C. Aspirin 300 mg od
D. Aspirin 300 mg od + dipyridamole 25 mg tds
E. No drug treatment recommended until after CT scan

73–78. Hormone replacement therapy

A. Combined oestrogen/progesterone
B. Continuous combined HRT
C. Oestradiol patches 50 μg
D. Oestradiol pessary
E. Raloxifene
F. Tibolone

For each of the patients below select from the list of options above the **single** most appropriate treatment option:

73. A 50-year-old woman requests 'no period' HRT. She is 1 year postmenopausal and also reports low libido and low mood.

74. A 60-year-old woman complains of atrophic vaginitis.

75. A 55-year-old woman requests HRT for hot flushes. She has had a hysterectomy.

76. A 50-year-old woman requests HRT but she does not want to see the return of her periods. She is 1 year postmenopausal.

77. A 60-year-old woman noted to have a kyphotic spine requests HRT.

78. A 40-year-old woman is confirmed to have premature menopause with elevated serum LH and FSH levels.

79–82. Dermatological conditions

A. Body lice
B. Contact dermatitis
C. Eczema
D. Leukoplakia
E. Lichen planus
F. Lichen sclerosus
G. Psoriasis
H. Scabies

For each of the patients below select from the list of options above the **single** most likely diagnosis:

79. A 40-year-old hairdresser presents with an itchy rash on her inner wrists. The lesions are small reddish-purple papules and appear in linear form.

80. An 80-year-old female resident of a nursing home presents with an itchy generalized rash over her body, which spares her face. She reports that the itching is worse at night. On examination she has an itchy papular rash with isolated vesicles on her hands.

81. A 50-year-old heavy smoker presents with a white lesion on the undersurface of his tongue.

82. A 28-year-old female who smokes 20 cigarettes per day presents with linear plaques and palmar pustulosis.

83–87. Match the following clinical scenarios with the appropriate timing of introduction of contraception after giving birth:

A. Immediately
B. Day 21
C. 4 weeks
D. 6 weeks
E. 8 weeks
F. Delayed until after baby's first birthday

83. A 35-year-old female decides she would like the progestogen-only pill form of contraception. She intends to breastfeed. She has no contraindications to the POP.

84. A 25-year-old female would like the Depo-Provera injection. She intends to breastfeed and has no contraindications to injectables.

85. A 44-year-old female would like sterilization after the birth of her 6th child.

86. A 40-year-old female would like the Mirena IUS fitted after the birth of her 3rd child.

87. A 30-year-old female would like to start Microgynon after giving birth. She intends to bottle-feed and has no contraindications to the COC.

88–96. National Service Framework for Coronary Heart Disease issued by the Department of Health

Fill in the spaces using the words from the list below:
A. I
B. V
C. North
D. South
E. African
F. Indian
G. Low-dose aspirin
H. Blood pressure
I. <130/80
J. <140/85
K. Statins
L. ACE inhibitors
M. Warfarin or aspirin
N. Beta-blockers
O. HbA1C
P. Spironolactone

CHD is the single commonest cause of premature death in the UK. Men of working age in social class _____ (88) are 50% more likely to die from CHD than men in the population as a whole. Death rates are higher for people living in the _____ (89) of the country. For people born in the _____ (90) subcontinent, the death rate from heart disease is 38% higher for men and 43% higher for women than rates for the country as a whole. People with diagnosed CHD or other occlusive arterial disease should be offered daily _____ (91) medication and advice and treatment to maintain a BP _____ (92). People who also have left ventricular dysfunction should be offered _____ (93). People who have also had an MI should be started on _____ (94). People over 60 years old who also have atrial fibrillation should commence _____ (95). Meticulous control of _____ (96) is advised for people who also have diabetes.

97–101. Match the following heart failure trials with their respective descriptions:

A. CIBIS II
B. CONSENSUS
C. ELITE
D. MERIT-HF
E. RALES
F. SOLVD

97. This study published in the *NEJM*, 1999, looked at a large RCT of people with NYHA class III/IV grade of heart failure on treatment including ACE inhibitors, and found that adding an aldosterone receptor antagonist (spironolactone) further decreased mortality.

98. This study published in the *Lancet* 1997 found that losartan in the elderly reduced symptoms of heart failure and mortality.

99. This trial published in the *Lancet* 1999 found that long-term use of beta-blockers, i.e. bisoprolol, in combination with ACE inhibitors in patients with NYHA class III/IV grade of heart failure reduced mortality.

100. This trial published in the *NEJM* in 2001 showed that adding enalapril in people on conventional treatment with NYHA class II/III heart failure improved symptoms, reduced mortality and reduced hospital admissions.

101. Published in the *Lancet* in 1999, this trial is the largest randomized, double-blind, placebo-controlled, multi-centred study of β_1-blockade in heart failure with 3991 patients treated. The study was conducted in 13 countries in Europe and the USA. This study showed that long-term use of metoprolol CR/XL, in addition to standard therapy including an ACE inhibitor, reduced total mortality and hospitalization by 31% in people with symptoms compatible with NYHA class II/III.

102–110. GP fees and allowances and superannuation

Match the following services with the appropriate payment category:

A. Capitation fees
B. Items of service payments
C. Practice allowances
D. Private medical work
E. Reimbursement

102. Contraceptive service fee

103. Maternity medical services (MMS)

104. Rural practice payments

105. Dispensing payments

106. Initial practice allowance

107. Childhood immunizations

108. Night visit payments

109. Cremation fees

110. Child health surveillance fee

111–115. Squint

Match the following definitions with the correct type of squint:

A. Esotropia
B. Exotropia
C. Latent squint
D. Paralytic
E. Pseudosquint

111. This is the commonest type in children and may be due to hypermetropia. Amblyopia may be a problem. One eye is turned in (convergent).

112. This is often intermittent and tends to occur in older children. Amblyopia is unlikely. One eye is turned out.

113. Diplopia is most marked when trying to look in the direction of the pull of the affected muscle.

114. Prominent epicanthal folds with a central and symmetrical corneal reflection from a bright light.

115. This squint is demonstrated by movement of the covered eye as the cover is removed during the cover test.

116–124. Types of study designs

Fill in the spaces using the appropriate word from the list below:

A. Cross-sectional
B. Case–control
C. Cohort
D. Randomized controlled
E. Null hypothesis
F. P-value
G. Odds ratio
H. Confidence interval
I. Confounding factor
J. Relative risk
K. Incidence

A _____ (**116**) study is a retrospective study that looks for exposure or presence of a factor association and not causation. It cannot calculate the incidence of a disease but can calculate the _____ (**117**) under certain conditions.

A _____ (**118**) study is a prospective study and can calculate incidence of disease directly, relative and attributable risk.

A _____ (**119**) study is descriptive in nature and provides a snapshot of the population in question. It cannot assess _____ (**120**).

A _____ (121) study gives the best evidence of cause and effect. It is an intervention study based on findings of observational studies.

A positive _____ (122) makes an association more extreme and leads to misleading association between two factors.

A narrow _____ (123) indicates less chance of sample variability and suggests greater certainty.

A _____ (124) of 1 indicates that there is no association between the exposure and the outcome.

125. Which of the following occupational chemical exposures are correctly linked with their respective diseases?
    A. Blue asbestos and lung cancer
    B. Cadmium and renal failure
    C. Fungal α-amylase and asthma
    D. Vinyl chloride and hepatic angiosarcoma
    E. Wood dust and sinonasal carcinoma

126. According to the 2003 British Thoracic Society/SIGN Guidelines on the treatment of asthma, step 3 following introduction of a short-acting β_2-agonist inhaler and regular low-dose inhaled steroids is:
    A. Add leukotriene receptor antagonist (LTRA)
    B. Add long-acting β_2-agonist
    C. Add SR theophylline
    D. Add trial course of oral steroids
    E. Double dose of inhaled steroids

127–131. Using the British Hypertension Society 1999 Guidelines for Management of Hypertension and NICE guidance June 2006, match the appropriate management option:
    A. Advise lifestyle changes and reassess monthly if 10-year CHD risk < 20%. Reassess CHD risk annually.
    B. If the 10-year CHD risk is ≥ 20%, target organ damage, CV complications or diabetes present, confirm over 12 weeks, then treat.
    C. Re-measure weekly if the 10-year CHD risk is < 20% with no target organ damage, CV complications or diabetes, and treat if these values are sustained on repeat measurements over 4–12 weeks.
    D. If the 10-year CHD risk is ≥ 20%, target organ damage, CV complications or diabetes present, confirm over 3–4 weeks then treat if these values are sustained.
    E. Regardless of 10-year CHD risk, confirm over 1–2 weeks then treat if these values are sustained.
    F. Regardless of 10-year CHD risk, confirm over 1–2 weeks then treat if these values are sustained. If malignant hypertension or hypertensive emergency, admit immediately.

127. A 65-year-old man is noted to have an initial BP of 220/100.

128. A 55-year-old woman is noted to have an initial BP of 170/100 but has no cardiovascular complications, end-organ damage or diabetes.

129. A 60-year-old man with type 2 diabetes is noted to have a BP of 150/95.

130. A 45-year-old man with LVH is noted to have a BP of 180/105.

131. A 40-year-old obese healthy woman is noted to have a BP of 150/90.

132–137. Evidence-based management of hypertension

    A. ACE inhibitor
    B. Alpha-blocker
    C. Angiotensin II receptor antagonists
    D. Beta-blocker
    E. Calcium antagonist (dihydropyridine)
    F. Calcium antagonists (rate-limiting)
    G. Thiazide diuretic

For each of the patients below select from the list of options above the **single** most appropriate antihypertensive drug, based on evidence:

132. A 75-year-old man with a history of gout is noted to have persistent BP > 170/80 over 3 months.

133. A 50-year-old Afro-Caribbean man requires antihypertensive therapy.

134. A 70-year-old man with a history of prostatism has a persistent BP > 170/100.

135. A 55-year-old man has a history of heart failure and requires antihypertensive therapy.

136. A 60-year-old woman on ramipril complains of persistent tickly cough.

137. A 65-year-old man with a history of angina is noted to have persistently elevated BP.

138–140. Match the following gynaecological cancers with the relevant risk age group:

A. Carcinoma of the body of the uterus
B. Carcinoma of the ovary
C. Cervical carcinoma
D. Vulval carcinoma

138. Age group 20–64 with a median age of 52 years

139. Over 40 with a median age of 60 years

140. Majority occurs in the 65–70 year-old age group

141, 142. If the incidence of DVT in a high-risk population of women aged 35–45 on combined desogestrel and ethinyoestradiol is 10%, and the incidence of DVT is 5% in a similar population of women who do not use the combined oral contraceptive pill, then what are the following values for:

141. Attributable risk

A. 1%
B. 2%
C. 5%
D. 10%
E. 15%
F. 25%

142. Numbers needed to treat

A. 10
B. 20
C. 25
D. 50
E. 100

143. Which of the following meningococcal vaccines is recommended for a family travelling to Saudi Arabia during the Haj pilgrimage?

A. Meningococcal Group C
B. Meningococcal Group A
C. Meningococcal Group AC
D. Meningococcal polysaccharide ACWY vaccine

144. The following symptoms may be associated with ricin (extract from beans of the castor oil plant):

A. Bloody diarrhoea
B. Cough
C. Fever
D. Heart failure
E. Seizure

145–148. Interpret the following spirometry test results and match to the most likely diagnosis:

A. FEV1/FVC = 76% with an FEV1 of 2.5 L
B. FEV1/FVC = 82% with an FEV1 of 1 L
C. FEV1/FVC = 40% with an FEV1 of 1.5 L

145. Severe emphysema

146. Extrinsic allergic alveolitis

147. Asthma

148. Sarcoidosis

149. The initial treatment for acute anaphylaxis is:

A. 0.5 ml of 1 : 1000 adrenaline IM
B. 0.5 ml of 1 : 1000 adrenaline IV
C. 0.5 ml of 1 : 1000 adrenaline SC
D. 0.5 ml of 1 : 10,000 adrenaline IM
E. 0.5 ml of 1 : 10,000 adrenaline IV

150–153. Confidence intervals/forest plots

Match the following statistical relevance with the confidence intervals depicted below:

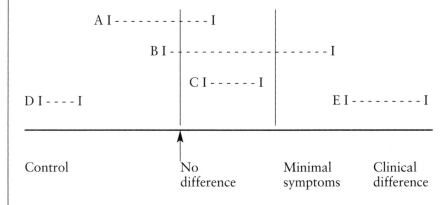

150. Statistically significant but with minimal symptoms

151. Not statistically significant and may be harmful

152. Statistically significant but not clinically significant

153. Clinically significant

154. If aspirin decreases the risk of cerebrovascular disease by 20%, then what is the relative risk of cerebrovascular disease in users of aspirin versus non-users?

A. 0.2
B. 0.4
C. 0.6
D. 0.8
E. 1.2

155. Relative risk is defined as:

A. The incidence of disease in the non-exposed population divided by the incidence of disease in the exposed population.
B. The incidence of disease in the non-exposed population minus the incidence of disease in the exposed population.
C. The incidence of disease in the exposed population divided by the incidence of disease in the non-exposed population
D. The incidence of disease in the exposed population minus the incidence of disease in the non-exposed population
E. The incidence of disease in the general population

156. Initial treatment for allergic nasal polyps as recommended in the *BNF* is:

A. Beconase nasal spray
B. Betnesol nasal drops
C. Prednisolone
D. Rynacrom nasal spray
E. Xylometazoline nasal drops

157. A 50-year-old woman is noted to have persistently elevated fasting blood glucose of > 7 mmol/L. She has a BMI of 31 and has tried to diet unsuccessfully. Which is the **single** most appropriate anti-diabetic drug for her?

A. Acarbose
B. Biguanide
C. Oral sulfonylurea
D. Repaglinide
E. Thiazolidinedione

158. A 65-year-old woman presents with myalgia. The serum full blood count is normal and the ESR comes back as 40 mm/h. The next step should be:

A. Arrange for CXR and AXR
B. Course of high-dose steroids as she most likely has polymyalgia rheumatica and cover with alendronate and lansoprazole
C. Reassurance
D. Refer for temporal artery biopsy
E. Take blood for CRP as it is more sensitive

159. The mother of an 8-year-old boy would like her son tested for allergy to peanuts as it runs in the family. Which **two** of the following investigations are the most appropriate? (Select **two** answers only.)

A. Nasal smear
B. Patch testing
C. RAST
D. Serum allergen specific IgE
E. Skin prick test

160. A 7-year-old boy presents with recurrent abdominal bloating, weight loss and diarrhoea. He is in the 5th percentile for height and weight. Which screening investigation is the **single** most sensitive?

A. Endomysial antibodies
B. Faecal fat estimation
C. Full blood count
D. Urea and electrolytes
E. Vitamin B_{12}/folate levels

161–164. Analgesia

A. Aspirin
B. Diamorphine
C. Diclofenac IM
D. Ibuprofen
E. Naratriptan
F. Paracetamol
G. Pizotifen
H. Tramadol PO

For each of the patients below select from the list of options above the **single** most appropriate type of analgesia:

161. A 45-year-old female presents with renal colic.

162. A 65-year-old man presents with severe angina and diaphoresis. BP is 90/50 mmHg. Pulse is 120 b/min.

163. A 60-year-old woman with metastatic breast cancer asks for analgesia for headaches.

164. A 30-year-old woman requests analgesia for migraines. She is on Prozac.

165. A 25-year-old woman states that she had her pill-free break but forgot to start a new pill pack on day 1. It is now day 2 and she has had UPSI yesterday. What is the **single** most appropriate management plan?

   A. Administer Levonelle-2.
   B. Offer an IUCD.
   C. Suggest she start the pack and omit the pill-free break.
   D. Take three pills today and resume pack as normal tomorrow.
   E. Wait until she sees her next period before starting the pill.

166. Which **three** of the following statements are true regarding the management of constipation in children:

   A. Abdominal x-ray must be obtained to exclude pathology.
   B. Evacuation of faecal impaction is offered under a GA.
   C. Faeces may be palpated in the abdomen.
   D. Lactulose may be prescribed.
   E. Rectal examination (PR) is often indicated to exclude faecal impaction.

167–171. Evidence-based management of LV dysfunction

   A. Amlodipine
   B. Diclofenac
   C. Digoxin
   D. Furosemide
   E. GTN
   F. Losartan
   G. Nicorandil
   H. Nifedipine
   I. Ramipril
   J. Spironolactone
   K. Verapamil
   L. Warfarin

Match the scenarios below with the drugs listed above:

167. A 60-year-old man is noted to have LV dysfunction on echo and a history of angina. From the list above, which **two** drugs are most appropriate in his management?

168. Which **two** drugs are contraindicated with LV dysfunction?

169. A 70-year-old man is noted to have LV dysfunction on echo and has an irregularly irregular pulse rate. From the list above, which **two** drugs should be added to his management?

170. A 65-year-old man is noted to have LV dysfunction and has fluid overload. Which **two** drugs should be offered in his management?

171. A 55-year-old man with LV dysfunction continues to have fluid overload and now has sodium retention despite thiazide diuretic, ramipril and bisoprolol. What should be added next?

172. Diagnosis of diabetes mellitus is best made by:

    A. Capillary sample
    B. Fasting blood glucose
    C. HbA1C
    D. Oral glucose tolerance test
    E. Random blood glucose

173–177. Haematological conditions

    A. Acute lymphoblastic leukaemia
    B. Acute myeloid leukaemia
    C. Chronic granulocytic leukaemia
    D. Chronic lymphocytic leukaemia
    E. Non-Hodgkin's lymphoma
    F. Hodgkin's disease
    G. Iron-deficiency anaemia
    H. Multiple myeloma
    I. Sickle-cell anaemia

For each of the patients below select from the list of options above the **single** most likely diagnosis:

173. A 14-year-old male presents with recurrent gum bleeding, sore throat, mouth ulcers and malaise. On examination he has a palpable spleen. Blood tests show elevated WCC with decreased platelets. Blood film shows a few blast cells. His father works in a gas station with regular exposure to petrol.

174. A 25-year-old female presents with an enlarged, painless cervical lymph node. She also reports drenching night sweats and has lost weight. Peripheral blood smear shows Reed–Sternberg cells with a bilobed, mirror-imaged nucleus.

175. A 70-year-old man presents with recurrent chest infections and chronic back pain. Blood tests reveal anaemia and elevated urea/creatinine. Blood tests reveal an elevated ESR and calcium. Bone marrow reveals an abundance of malignant plasma cells.

176. An 8-year-old boy presents with swelling of the hands and feet. Hb is 8 mg/dL. Peripheral blood smear reveals target cells and elongated crescent-shaped red blood cells.

177. A 65-year-old woman presents with dysphagia. She is also noted to have spoon-shaped fingernails and a smooth tongue. Blood smear reveals microcytic, hypochromic blood cells.

178–184. Algorithm for the management of jaundice

    A. Conjugated
    B. Unconjugated
    C. Gallstones present
    D. No gallstones present
    E. CT scan
    F. Ultrasound
    G. ERCP
    H. PTC
    I. Liver biopsy

Complete the gaps in the algorithm from the list above:

JAUNDICE

History, examination, urine and blood tests including viral markers

Raised plasma (178) _____ BR
Urinary urobilinogen increased

Raised plasma (179) _____ BR
No urinary urobilinogen

(180) _____

No dilatation of common bile duct

Dilatation of common bile duct

(181) _____ (182) _____

If PTC or ERCP is normal, then (183) _____

(184) _____ or surgery

185. A 20-year-old pregnant woman presents with asymptomatic bacteriuria. The most appropriate antibiotic regime is:

A. Cefadroxil 0.5 g–1 g bd × 3 days
B. Co-amoxyclavulanic acid 375 mg tds × 7 days
C. Nalidixic acid 1 g qds × 5 days
D. Nitrofurantoin 50 mg qds × 7 days
E. Trimethoprim 200 mg bd × 3 days

186. Risk factors for osteoporosis include:

A. Gastric surgery
B. Muslim female
C. Overexercise
D. Repeated short courses of steroids
E. Smoking

187–190. Match the following age groups with the appropriate recommended immunizations. There may be more than one recommended vaccine per age group:

A. Adult DT
B. Polio
C. MMR
D. HiBDPT
E. Men C

187. At 2, 3, and 4 months of age

188. 12–15 months of age

189. 3–4 year-olds (preschool)

190. 14–18 year-olds

191–194. Urinary incontinence

    A. Cystocoele
    B. Disc prolapse
    C. Multiple sclerosis
    D. Pelvic floor prolapse
    E. Senile vaginitis
    F. Urinary tract infection
    G. Vesico-vaginal fistula

For each of the patients below select from the list of options above the **single** most likely diagnosis:

191. A 55-year-old woman reports persistent urinary incontinence post vaginal hysterectomy.

192. A 60-year-old-man presents with back pain. On examination, he has saddle anaesthesia, urinary incontinence and loss of anal tone.

193. A 70-year-old woman reports 3 months of urinary incontinence. She is ashamed to bring this up with you. Coughing makes matters worse. MSU is normal.

194. A 40-year-old woman presents with double vision, weakness in both legs and urinary incontinence.

195–200. Childhood illnesses

    A. Appendicitis
    B. Bronchiolitis
    C. Gastroenteritis
    D. Hand-foot-and-mouth disease
    E. Henoch–Schönlein purpura
    F. Kawasaki's disease
    G. Meningococcal septicaemia
    H. Pneumonia

For each of the patients below select from the list of options above the **single** most likely diagnosis:

195. A 13-year-old girl presents with a non-blanching rash and drowsiness.

196. A 10-year-old boy presents with a haemorrhagic purpuric rash over the lower half of his body.

197. An 8-year-old girl presents with fever, polymorphous rash, lip fissuring and erythema of the hands and feet.

198. An 18-month-old baby presents with fever and vomiting. The ears, throat and chest exams are normal.

199. A 2-month-old baby presents with wheeze and cough. On exam, basal creps are auscultated.

200. A 3-year-old girl presents with spiking fever, dry cough, left shoulder tip pain and left upper abdominal pain.

Applied Knowledge Test Module Paper One: Answers

1. ABCDE. Asplenia or severe dysfunction of the spleen, including homozygous sickle cell disease and coeliac syndrome, chronic heart disease, chronic liver disease, including cirrhosis, chronic lung disease, diabetes mellitus, chronic renal disease or nephrotic syndrome, immunodeficiency or immunosuppression due to disease or treatment, including HIV at all stages, are all indications for pneumococcal vaccination. The MDA Agency Advice, August 2002, includes unvaccinated cochlear implant patients.

2. ABCDE. Viagra is licensed for ED in men who have DM, MS, Parkinson's, poliomyelitis, prostate cancer, severe pelvic injury, spina bifida, spinal cord injury, or who have had radical pelvic surgery, prostatectomy or kidney transplant.

3. A. The incus is one of the three middle ear bones. Behind this sits the stapes (stirrup).

4. C. The manubrium of the malleus. The malleus is the most anterior bone.

5. D. The pars flaccida is the attic region of the eardrum and where we look for cholesteatoma (overgrowth of squamous cell debris).

6. E. The pars tensa is the area of the eardrum below the pars flaccida (attic).

7. B. The light reflex reflects light in the antero-inferior part of the eardrum.

8. C. At 6 months, a baby can sit with support, transfer a cube from hand to hand and shows person preference.

9. E. By 8 months, a baby can sit without support.

10. L. A 5-year-old child can hop on one foot, count 10–12 objects, knows 3–4 colours and shows friend preference.

11. A. A 6-week-old baby can track an object 1 m away, smile, startle and has both a Moro and a grasp reflex.

12. H. By 18 months, a baby can build a 3–4-cube tower, speak 10–12 words, ask for a potty, use a spoon and jump with both feet.

13. K. A 4-year-old child can copy a circle and a cross, use a tricycle, catch a ball and knows his or her first and last names.

14. B. A 12-week-old baby can turn his or her head to sounds at the level of the ear. By 7 months, a baby can turn his or her head to sounds below the level of the ear.

15. A. However, if the driver was diagnosed with AIDS syndrome, revocation of the licence is recommended for group 2 entitlement.

16. H. Stable/unstable angina requires a ban on driving if angina occurs at rest or at the wheel. For HGV drivers (group 2), revocation is recommended; however, re-licensing can occur if the driver has been symptom-free for 6/52 and passes the exercise stress test criteria.

17. D. A first fit associated with misuse of alcohol or drugs or a neurosurgical condition requires a ban on driving for at least 1 year with medical review before restarting driving.

18. B

19. B. Any cerebrovascular condition, e.g. stroke due to TIA, amaurosis fugax, intracerebral haemorrhage, requires a ban on driving for at least 1 month. For group 2 entitlement the ban is for 1 year.

20. C. Current recommendations suggest permethrin or malathion as first-line treatment for scabies. Hot baths have now been found to increase absorption of topical treatment into the bloodstream away from the site of action, i.e. the skin. All members of the affected household should be treated.

21. E

22. A

23. B

24. C

25. F

26. H

27. F

28. D

29. C

30. A

31. G

32. B

33. I

34. J

35. C

36. H

37. G

38. F

39. D

40. A

41. ABCDE

42. B

43. ABDE. Urgent referral is recommended for painless macroscopic haematuria in adults.

44. ABCDE

45. C. Cervical screening is three-yearly between ages 25 and 49 and five-yearly between ages 50 and 64.

46. E

47. E. Otosclerosis often presents in pregnancy and may be associated with normal TMs and blue sclerae.

48. F. Presbyacusis or old age hearing loss. Hearing aids are fitted when hearing is diminished in the low frequency range, i.e. range for TV, radio, phone, conversation.

49. B

50. C

51. A. These symptoms warrant an MRI of the internal acoustic meati to exclude acoustic neuroma.

52. A

53. D

54. C

55. B

56. E

57. C

58. G

59. D

60. A

61. F

62. E

63. ABCD. Domiciliary oxygen is recommended for patients with pulmonary malignancy or other terminal disease with disabling dyspnoea.

64. ABCDEF. Pregnant women should avoid basil, cedarwood, clary sage, juniper berry, marjoram, myrrh and sage. Patients with epilepsy should avoid fennel, sage and rosemary. Hypertensive patients should avoid rosemary, sage, thyme and stimulating spice oils. Citrus oils and bergamot should be avoided prior to sun exposure. Patients using homeopathy should then avoid camphor, chamomile and mint oils as these may neutralize the effects of homeopathy; and finally skin testing should be performed to assess allergy or skin irritation.

65. A

66. ABDE. In August 2005, the *Lancet* published a paper that disproved homeopathy once and for all, looking at 110 RCTs comparing homeopathy with conventional medicine and proved that homeopathy had the same efficacy rate as the placebo effect. The placebo effect was proven by HK Beecher.

67. D

68. F

69. C

70. B

71. A

72. B

73. F   Tibolone is androgenic.

74. D

75. C

76. B

77. E

78. A

79. E

80. H

81. D

82. G

83. B

84. D.   Six weeks is advised to allow the baby's liver enzymes to mature.

85. F

86. D

87. B

88. B

89. C

90. F

91. G

92. J

93. L

94. N

95. M

96. H

97. E

98. C

99. A

100. F

101. D

102. B.   Items of service payments include night visits, emergency treatment, immediately necessary treatment, cervical cytology fee, contraceptive fee, anaesthetic fee, dental haemorrhage fee, health promotion fees, immunizations, maternity fees, and minor op fees.

103. B

104. C. Practice allowances include absence allowances to cover locums, study leave, PGEA course, confinement, etc., assistant or associate's allowances, basic and initial practice allowances, designated area allowance and rural practice payment.

105. E. Reimbursement includes GO computer reimbursement scheme, dispensing fees, out-of-hours development scheme, practice staff scheme and reimbursement of rent, rates and sewerage.

106. C

107. B

108. B

109. D. Private medical work includes reports for insurance companies, solicitors, lecturing, fitness to drive, HGV licence, court witness, cremation fees and other private medical exams.

110. A. Capitation fees include standard capitation fee for patients aged < 65, 65–74, and 75 and over, child health surveillance, deprivation payments, registration fee, and temporary resident fees.

111. A

112. B

113. D

114. E

115. C. All squints require ophthamological assessment. Management is divided into the 3 'O's: optical, orthoptic and operation. The refractive state of the eyes is determined after use of mydriatic eye drops, and the eyes are inspected to exclude cataract, macular scarring, optic atrophy, retinoblastoma, etc. Spectacles are offered to correct any refractive errors. Orthoptic is the patching of the good eye to encourage use of the squinting (lazy) eye. Finally resection and recession of the rectus muscles is reserved for cosmesis or alignment.

116. B

117. G

118. C

119. A

120. K

121. D

122. I

123. H

124. J

125. ABCDE.   Commercial bakers are exposed to fungal amylase additives to flour, which cause occupational asthma. Cadmium is also associated with respiratory disease.

126. B.   Guidelines have recently been changed as of February 2003. The addition of long-acting β_2-agonists is now advocated, prior to increasing the dose of inhaled steroids to 800 µg/day. If there is no response to an inhaled LABA + increased steroid, then an LTRA or SR theophylline is introduced. Step 4 is as before, increasing the inhaled steroids to 2000 µg/day and possibly adding an LTRA. Step 5 is the introduction of daily oral steroids and referral of the patient for specialist care.

127. F

128. C

129. B

130. D

131. A

132. E

133. G

134. B

135. A

136. C

137. D

138. C. Cervical cancer is the second most common malignancy after breast cancer. The relevant risk age corresponds to the target age for cervical smear screening.

139. A. Carcinoma of the body of the uterus is less frequent than cancer of the cervix or ovary.

140. D

141. C. Attributable risk is the incidence in the exposed population minus the incidence in the non-exposed population.

142. B   NNT=1/ARR%= 1/ (% treated group with desired outcome minus % controls with desired outcome).

143. D. 35 deaths have occurred during the Haj pilgrimage of 2001 with > 100 cases of W135 serotype meningococcal meningitis. For 2003, the Hajj will take place in the first week of March. Outside the Haj and Umrah pilgrimages, Men A&C vaccination is adequate and also recommended for travel in other areas of risk, i.e. Nepal, Pakistan, Bhutan and the meningitis belt of Africa.

144. ABCDE.   Ricin is 6000 times more lethal than cyanide per gram. There is no cure and treatment is supportive. Symptoms may surface between 1–7 days following exposure by inhalation, ingestion or injection. Ingestion of 8 seeds is lethal in an adult.

145. C.   In obstructive disease, the FEV1/FVC ratio < 80% with an FEV1 of
          < 80% predicted. In restrictive disease, the FEV1/FVC ratio > 80% with
          an FEV1 of < 80% predicted. Normally, the FEV1 should be > 80% pre-
          dicted with an FEV1/FVC ratio between 70% and 80%.

146. B

147. A

148. B

149. A

150. B

151. A

152. C

153. E

154. D.   The relative risk in this case is calculated as 1 − (20% of 1) = 0.8.

155. C.   Option D is the definition of attributable risk and option E the def-
          inition of absolute risk. Know how to calculate relative risk and NNR for
          the exam (popular question).

156. B

157. B

158. C.   The upper limits of normal for ESR = (10 + age) divided by 2. This
          woman's ESR is normal but you may wish to repeat in 6 months. Alarm
          bells should ring if the ESR was > 100 mm/h. Causes of elevated ESR
          include rheumatoid arthritis, infection, malignancy, connective tissue dis-
          orders (giant cell arteritis), sarcoidosis, and renal disease.

159. DE. Skin prick testing should be conducted in a specialist chest clinic as there is a high risk of anaphylaxis.

160. A

161. C

162. B. Although you would also give aspirin while awaiting the ambulance.

163. H

164. E

165. C

166. BCD. It is rare to subject a child to a PR examination. Firm stool should be palpable during abdominal examination.

167. AE

168. BK

169. CL

170. DI

171. J

172. B. A FBG > 7 confirms diabetes. If the FBG is borderline (between 7 and 8), do an oral glucose tolerance test. The OGTT should normally be < 7.8 at 2 hours postprandial.

173. A

174. F

175. H

176. I

177. G

178. B

179. A

180. F

181. D

182. C

183. I

184. G

185. A.   50% of *E. coli* is now resistant to ampicillin.

186. ABCE.   Other risk factors include excessive alcohol, repeated steroid use in inflammatory bowel disease, family history, inactivity, lack of oestrogen and low testosterone in men.

187. BDE

188. C

189. CD

190. AB

191. G

192. B

193. D

194. C

195. G

196. E

197. F

198. C

199. B

200. H.   Left-sided basal pneumonia can present in children with left-sided abdominal pain with referred shoulder tip pain from irritation of the diaphragm via the phrenic nerve.

Applied Knowledge Test Module Paper Two: Questions

1–5. Match the following antihypertensive drugs with their noted side effects. There may be more than one answer:

A. ACE inhibitor
B. Alpha-blocker
C. Angiotensin receptor antagonist
D. Beta-blocker
E. Calcium antagonist
F. Diuretic

1. Cold hands and feet

2. Stress incontinence

3. Headache

4. Flushing

5. Impotence

6. The following statements are **true** concerning case–control studies:

A. They can prove causation.
B. They cannot calculate risk ratio.
C. They are particularly useful for investigating rare diseases.
D. They are expensive to conduct.
E. They are retrospective.

7. A 60-year-old woman sustains a hip fracture. Upon discharge from hospital, you decide to put her on medication for osteoporosis. Besides, Calcichew D3 Forte, you should add which **single** medication:

A. Alendronic acid
B. Calcitonin
C. Raloxifene
D. HRT
E. Tiludronic acid

8. **Four** contraindications to the use of nicotine replacement therapy include:

   A. Breastfeeding
   B. Chronic psoriasis
   C. Diabetes mellitus
   D. Recent TIA
   E. Severe cardiovascular disease

9. Which **three** statements are true concerning anthrax?

   A. CXR findings are classic for anthrax.
   B. Ciprofloxacin is the antibiotic of choice.
   C. Contacts of exposed individuals require prophylaxis.
   D. ID50 is the dose required to infect 50% of exposed individuals.
   E. It is a notifiable disease.

10. Which of the following diseases are notifiable to the Consultant in Communicable Disease Control (Multiple Best Answer (MBA))?

    A. Cholera
    B. Food poisoning
    C. Measles
    D. Scarlet fever
    E. Viral hepatitis

11. A 13-month-old baby presents with a 36-hour history of right earache and high fever. On exam, $T = 39°C$ and the tympanic membrane is red and bulging. The most appropriate treatment is (**single best answer**):

    A. Amoxicillin
    B. Ibuprofen
    C. Paracetamol
    D. Reassurance and review
    E. Calpol

12. The following **four** statements are true regarding coronary heart disease and air travel: (Source: *OHGP*)

    A. A symptom-free patient following coronary angioplasty is fit to travel after 2 weeks.
    B. If a patient with LVF requires oxygen at rest, flying is contraindicated.
    C. If a patient with coronary heart disease cannot manage a flight of stairs without stopping he/she is not fit for flying.
    D. There need be no bar with unstable angina.
    E. Travel should be delayed for 3 weeks following a recent myocardial infarction.

13. The **single** most common presentation of stroke is:

   A. Aphasia
   B. Dysphagia
   C. Loss of consciousness
   D. Sudden onset of hemiplegia
   E. Sudden visual field deficit

14. The following statements are **true** regarding evidence-based management of stroke (MBA):

   A. Aspirin 300 mg should be started within 48 hours of a haemorrhagic stroke.
   B. Thombolysis is offered routinely.
   C. Heparin prophylaxis is indicated if the patient has morbid obesity.
   D. Heparin is indicated for recurrent embolic TIAs.
   E. DVT and PE develop in 50% of patients after an ischaemic stroke.

15–19. Statin trials

   A. AFCAPS/TexCaps, *JAMA*
   B. CARE, *NEJM*, 1996
   C. 4S Trial, *Lancet* 1994
   D. Heart protection study, *Lancet* 2002
   E. WOSCOPS
   F. LIPID study, *NEJM* 1998

   Match the following study descriptions with their correlating trials listed above:

15. This study showed the benefits of reducing cholesterol in healthy men and women with average cholesterol levels.

16. This 5-year, randomized, controlled study of 20,536 individuals with cardiac disease or diabetes showed that 40 mg of simvastatin reduced the risk of MI, stroke and revascularization by one-third, even in patients with normal or low blood cholesterol levels.

17. This was a prospective trial of 4,444 patients with coronary heart disease and raised cholesterol. This trial showed a reduction of relative risk of coronary mortality of 42% in patients treated with simvastatin 20–40 mg a day. Greatest benefit was achieved in patients > 60 years of age or patients with DM.

18. This randomized trial of 6,595 middle-aged men with mean cholesterol of 7 mmol/L showed a 31% reduction in coronary mortality in those treated with 40 mg pravastatin a day and a 20% reduction in cholesterol in the treated group.

19. This randomized, controlled trial of 4,159 men and women aged 21–75 years who had suffered an MI in the past 2 years and had an average total cholesterol of 5.4 mmol/L were randomized to pravastatin or placebo and followed at 5 years. The study showed that reducing cholesterol level with pravastatin after MI reduced risk of CHD death/non-fatal MI by 24%, of fatal MI by 37% and of stroke by 28%.

20. The following statements are **true** concerning renal medicine:

   A. Orthostatic proteinuria in an adolescent with a total daily protein excretion of < 1g may be ignored.
   B. Patients < 40 with microscopic haematuria and hypertension should be referred to a nephrologist.
   C. Patients with a serum creatinine > 150 µmol/L should be referred to a nephrologist.
   D. Patients with type 1 diabetes and repeated microalbuminuria should be commenced on an ACE inhibitor.
   E. Renal function should be checked at initiation and 2–3 weeks after starting or increasing an ACE inhibitor or angiotensin receptor II inhibitor.

21. The following statements are **true** concerning drug therapy for obesity:

   A. According to NICE guidelines, patients must have a BMI > 30 kg/m^2 and no longer need to have produced a weight loss > 2.5 kg over 4 weeks before commencing orlistat.
   B. Orlistat acts by inhibiting the action of pancreatic lipase, thus reducing the digestion and absorption of dietary fat.
   C. Pulse and blood pressure must be monitored frequently prior to and during treatment with orlistat.
   D. Sibutramine acts by promoting and prolonging satiety after eating.
   E. Side effects of sibutramine include fatty oily stool.

22–25. Orthopaedic conditions

A. Calcaneal stress fracture
B. Osgood-Schlatter disease
C. Patello-femoral syndrome
D. Patellar tendinitis
E. Plantar fasciitis

For each of the patients below select the **single** most likely diagnosis from the above list of options:

22. A 40-year-old woman complains of heel pain. Pain is worse putting the heel onto the floor in the morning but eases as she walks. On examination she has point tenderness 4 cm forward from the heel.

23. A 20-year-old woman presents with heel pain. She enjoys running in marathons. Pain is elicited on squeezing the lateral aspect of the calcaneus.

24. A 25-year-old ballet dancer reports anterior knee pain with clicking and crepitus of the knee. On examination, she has medial patellar tenderness and a mild effusion.

25. A 14-year-old girl reports anterior knee pain. On examination the tibial tubercle is prominent and tender.

26–31. Eye conditions

A. Acute conjunctivitis
B. Acute iritis
C. Central retinal artery occlusion
D. Central retinal vein occlusion
E. Closed angled glaucoma
F. Posterior communicating aneurysm
G. Retinal detachment
H. Vitreous haemorrhage

26. An 8-year-old child presents with sudden diplopia, ptosis and a lateral diverging eye.

27. A 60-year-old woman complains of a 'curtain coming down' over her right eye with painless loss of vision. She mentions seeing flashing lights first.

28. A 40-year-old man complains of a painful red eye with photophobia and pain on accommodation. The pupil is irregular.

29. A 70-year-old woman presents with a cloudy cornea, reduced visual acuity and painful red eye.

30. A 75-year-old woman presents with sudden loss of vision in the left eye with acuity reduced to finger counting. The fundus resembles a bloodstorm!

31. A 60-year-old woman presents with sudden loss of vision in the right eye with acuity reduced to light perception. The retina appears white with a cherry-red spot on the macula. She comments that she had transient blindness before full blindness of the right eye.

32–34. ECGs

A. Acute myocardial infarction
B. Acute pericarditis
C. Pulmonary embolus

Match the following descriptions of ECG abnormalities with the correct diagnosis from the list above.

32. Q-waves in leads II, III, avF with ST-elevation and T-wave inversion.

33. Deep S-waves in lead I, pathological Q-waves in III and inverted T-wave in lead III.

34. Concave, saddle-shaped ST-segment elevation.

35. The following statements are **true** concerning heart failure:

A. NICE recommendations 2003 suggest GPs use a blood test for the marker N-terminal pro-brain natriuretic peptide (NT-proBNP) to exclude heart failure.
B. Echocardiogram is the gold standard for diagnosing heart failure.
C. Angiotensin receptor blockers are a first-line therapy in chronic heart failure.
D. Spironolactone should be added to patients in advanced heart failure (NYHA class III/IV).
E. Beta-blockers are associated with deterioration in the patient's quality of life during the first 3 months of therapy.

36. Which **one** of the following should be suggested for a baby with intractable colic?

   A. Soya milk
   B. Sugared water
   C. Anticholinergic drugs
   D. Infacol
   E. Gripe water

37–42. Laboratory investigations

   A. ESR
   B. Ferritin
   C. Platelets
   D. Serum protein electrophoresis
   E. Vitamin B_{12}
   F. White blood count

For each of the patients below select the **single** most discriminating investigation from the above list of options.

37. A 40-year-old man post gastrectomy presents with anaemia.

38. A 30-year-old woman with a history of fibroids presents with angular cheilosis.

39. A 20-year-old woman presents with recurrent epistaxis, easy bruisability and heavy periods.

40. A 35-year-old man presents with chronic fatigue and shortness of breath with mild exertion. He is also noted to have bronzed skin and arthralgia of the MCP joints.

41. A 10-year old boy presents with a purple rash on his buttocks that does not disappear on pressure.

42. A 70-year-old man presents with a compression fracture of his spine.

43. According to the NICE guidelines for the management of type 2 diabetes the following statements are **true**:

   A. Aim for blood pressure < 140/80 mmHg.
   B. Patients who do not have manifest cardiovascular disease should have their heart disease risk estimated annually.
   C. Patients whose blood pressure is found to be > 160/100 mmHg should be treated with ACE inhibitors.
   D. Patients with type 2 diabetes should be tested annually for microalbuminuria.
   E. Patients with type 2 diabetes should have annual serum fasting lipids.

44. According to evidence-based medicine, the **single** most appropriate step to take in management of a male patient noted to have a total cholesterol of 6.0 mmol/L, LDL-C 3.5 mmol/L and TG of 2 mmol/L is:

   A. Assess coronary heart disease risk.
   B. Commence fibrate.
   C. Commence simvastatin 40 mg nocte.
   D. Offer dietary advice.
   E. Refer to specialist lipid clinic.

45. A 50 year-old woman reports night sweats and hot flushes. Which blood test would you order to confirm menopause?

   A. FSH
   B. LH
   C. Progesterone
   D. Prolactin
   E. Testosterone

46. The Royal College of Physicians suggest that bone mineral density measurements should be offered to the following groups of patients:

   A. Radiographic evidence of vertebral deformity
   B. Body mass index < 19 kg/m^2
   C. Prednisolone > 7.5 mg daily for 6 months or more
   D. Premature menopause (age < 45 years)
   E. Maternal history of hip fracture

47. An 8-year-old girl presents with 3 days of fever, sore throat and generalized lymphadenopathy. FBC reveals raised WCC, mostly atypical lymphocytes and mildly elevated ALT. Monospot test comes back as negative. The **single** most appropriate step is:

A. Arrange for immunofluorescence test for EBV-specific IgM.
B. Arrange for liver scan.
C. Repeat monospot test.
D. Reassure patient that she does not have glandular fever.
E. Take throat swab for *Streptococcus*.

48. The **single** most appropriate treatment for senile watery rhinorrhoea is:

A. Betnesol nasal drops
B. Sodium cromoglycate
C. Sympathomimetic drug, e.g. pseudoephedrine
D. Topical antihistamine nasal spray, e.g. Rhinolast
E. Topical nasal ipratropium spray, e.g. Rinatec

49. Recognized treatments for nasal polyps include all of the following **except**:

A. Betnesol nasal drops
B. Functional endoscopic sinus surgery (FESS)
C. Oral corticosteroids
D. Snare polypectomy
E. Topical nasal ipratropium spray

50. Recognized treatments of severe symptomatic pulmonary hypertension include:

A. Bosentan (orally active non-selective antagonist of endothelin)
B. Calcium channel blockers
C. Heart–lung transplantation
D. Prostacyclin (Epoprostenol) infusion
E. Regular nebulization of Iloprost

51. Select the **single** most appropriate drug treatment for depression in the elderly:

A. Donepezil
B. Dothiepin
C. Moclobemide
D. Sertraline
E. Venlafaxine

52. A 40-year-old mature student is diagnosed with schizophrenia. His acute psychosis is managed in hospital. Upon discharge, he should be maintained on:

A. Clozapine
B. Haloperidol
C. Olanzapine
D. Piportal
E. Risperidone

53–57. Urinanalysis

A. RBC > 300/mm³, WBC 100/mm³, no organisms
B. RBC 100/mm³, WBC 100/mm³, no organisms
C. RBC 50/mm³, WBC < 10/mm³, no organisms
D. RBC < 10/mm³, WBC 100/mm³, *E. coli* growth, urine specific gravity 1.025
E. No RBCs, no WBC, urine specific gravity 1.002

Match the urinanalysis reports with the **single** most likely diagnosis from the list below:

53. Acute pyelonephritis

54. Bladder carcinoma

55. Diabetes insipidus

56. Renal calculus

57. Renal tuberculosis

58. Select **two** best answers for the treatment of scabies (*BNF*):

A. Apply cream twice, 1 week apart.
B. Hot bath before treatment application.
C. Treat all members of the household.
D. Wash all bedding in boiling water.
E. Wash curtains and steam-clean carpets.

59. Select **two** correct statements regarding the spread and treatment of clothing lice:

    A. They can walk from person to person.
    B. Lice can survive if clothes are not worn for 3 days or more.
    C. Live on the hair and body.
    D. Require treatment with insecticides.
    E. Wash clothes in water > 60°C.

60–65. Contraception

    A. IUCD
    B. Mirena
    C. Levonelle-2
    D. Depo-Provera injections
    E. POP
    F. Combined oral contraceptive
    G. Condom
    H. Norethisterone
    I. Lactational amenorrhoea method (LAM)
    J. Sterilization

For each of the patients below select the **single** most appropriate form of contraception from the above list of options:

60. A 40-year-old woman with a history of menorrhagia requests contraception. She is forgetful, very busy and hates needles. She does not plan on having any more children.

61. A 20-year-old woman requests contraception. She had UPSI on day 12 of her cycle, which was 2 days ago. She was not on any form of contraception.

62. A 30-year-old woman requests a pill to help her stop her periods while she is holidaying in Corsica.

63. A 32-year-old woman with a history of polycystic ovarian disease requests contraception.

64. A 25-year-old woman with multiple sexual partners requests contraception. She smokes 40 cigarettes a day and her BMI is > 30. She has had two abortions in the past.

65. A 30-year-old woman 4 weeks postpartum requests contraception. She is breastfeeding and has not had a period.

66–70. Analgesia

A. Bisphosphonates
B. COX-2 inhibitors
C. Futuro splint
D. Local steroid injection
E. Methotrexate
F. NSAIDs
G. Tramadol

For each of the patients below select the **single** most appropriate form of analgesia from the above list of options:

66. A 25-year-old pregnant woman complains of numbness and tingling in the thumb, index and middle fingers of her right hand that is worse at night.

67. A 50-year-old woman with metastatic breast carcinoma complains of headaches.

68. A 55-year-old woman presents with a hot and swollen MT joint. She has had no relief with paracetamol. She has no history of peptic ulcer disease.

69. A 65-year-old woman suffers from disabling rheumatoid arthritis of the hands, wrists and right knee. She also has active peptic ulcer disease and heart failure.

70. A 40-year-old carpenter presents with pain on the lateral aspect of his elbow. He reports that the pain is worse when he uses his screwdriver. You suspect tennis elbow. What is the **single** definitive treatment?

71. The **single** best cleaning agent for contaminated body fluids on work surfaces is:

A. Betadine
B. Chlorhexidine
C. Hypochlorite
D. Sodium chloride
E. Sodium perborate

72. A 30-year-old woman is found to have positive antiphospholipid antibody following a first-trimester miscarriage. She is at risk of:

   A. Arterial thrombosis
   B. Deep venous thrombosis
   C. Multi-infarct dementia
   D. Pre-eclampsia
   E. Stroke

73. Which drugs cause gout?

   A. Aspirin
   B. Ciclosporin
   C. Ethambutol
   D. Loop diuretic
   E. Nicotinic acid
   F. Pyrazinamide

74–77. Investigations for jaundice

   A. ERCP
   B. Liver biopsy
   C. Liver ultrasound
   D. Percutaneous transhepatic cholangiography
   E. Serum antimitochondrial antibodies
   F. Viral serology

   For each of the patients below select the **single** most discriminating investigation from the above list of options:

74. A 30-year-old business man returns from a trip to the Far East and complains of anorexia, malaise, pale stools and dark urine.

75. A 45-year-old woman presents with a 3-year history of jaundice, pruritus, pale stools and dark urine.

76. A 40-year-old man presents with jaundice and malaise. His ferritin level is high and his LFTs are mildly elevated. He does not drink alcohol.

77. A 60-year-old man presents with jaundice, pale stools and dark urine following laparoscopic cholecystectomy. Ultrasound reveals dilated common bile duct.

78–83. Respiratory conditions

A. Amoxicillin
B. Clarithromycin
C. Losartan
D. Prednisolone
E. Ramipril
F. Salbutamol inhaler

For each of the patients below select the **single** most appropriate treatment option from the above list of options:

78. A 50-year-old farmer presents with sudden onset of dry cough, fever and shortness of breath. Chest exam reveals basal crackles.

79. A 55-year-old man presents with cough, orthopnoea and paroxysmal nocturnal dyspneoa. On examination, he has a raised JVP and basal rales on auscultation.

80. A 30-year-old man presents with nocturnal cough. His FEV1 is 70% of predicted.

81. A 20-year-old man presents with swinging fever, non-productive cough and tender subcutaneous nodules on his anterior legs.

82. A 60-year-old woman on ramipril develops a tickly cough. Chest exam is normal.

83. A 50-year-old homeless man smelling of alcohol presents with fever and a productive cough. Chest exam reveals coarse rhonchi.

84–90. Fitness to drive (www.dvla.gov.uk)

A. No driving licence restrictions
B. 1 month off driving
C. 6 months off driving
D. 12 months off driving
E. Disqualified from driving until treated
F. Permanently barred and requires DVLA notification
G. Refusal or revocation
H. Driving must cease until cause identified
I. Relicensing when symptom-free for 6/52

Match the following scenarios with the appropriate fitness-to-drive regulations:

84. A man reaches his 70th birthday and denies medical disability.

85. A 50-year-old red bus driver has a persistent BP of 180/100 mmHg.

86. A 60-year-old man is diagnosed with metastatic carcinoma of the lung with secondaries in the bone and brain.

87. A 40-year-old man has an acute subdural haematoma requiring burr holes to evacuate.

88. A 30-year-old man has colour blindness and a visual acuity of 6/9 in both eyes.

89. A 20-year-old IVDA heroin misuser tests positive for opiates in his urine. He would like to initiate methadone treatment.

90. A 35-year old HGV driver reports that he faints at the sight of blood.

91–95. Glomerulopathy

A. IgA nephropathy
B. Minimal change glomerulonephritis
C. Henoch–Schönlein purpura
D. Thin membrane nephropathy
E. Focal segmental glomerulosclerosis
F. Mesangiocapillary glomerulonephritis
G. Membranous nephropathy
H. Proliferative GN
I. Rapidly progressive GN

For each of the patients below select the **single** most likely diagnosis from the above list of options:

91. A 4-year-old boy presents with proteinuria, oedema and hypoalbuminuria. Renal biopsy shows fusion of podocytes on electron microscopy.

92. A 20-year-old man with HIV presents with nephrotic syndrome and hypertension. Renal biopsy shows hyalinization of glomerular capillaries and positive IF for IgM and C3.

93. A 35-year-old woman with SLE presents with renal impairment. Renal biopsy reveals thickened BM, IF positive for IgG and C3, and subepithelial deposits on EM.

94. An 80-year-old woman presents with loin pain, haematuria and fever. She was well 1 month prior. Her ESR is elevated and she has fundoscopic features of giant cell arteritis. Renal biopsy reveals a focal necrotizing GN with crescent formation.

95. A 10-year-old boy with sickle cell disease presents with features of nephrotic syndrome. Renal biopsy reveals large glomeruli with double BM and subendothelial deposits.

96. Which **three** statements are correct regarding recent evidence on HRT?

    A. According to the HERS (Heart and Estrogen/Progestin Replacement Study), the absolute risk for VTE per 100,000 women per year was 620 in HRT users and 230 in non-HRT users.
    B. According to the WHI (Women's Health Initiative) study, for every 10,000 person-years there were seven more CHD events and eight more strokes than in the non-HRT group.
    C. Raloxifene is useful in the management of menopausal symptoms.
    D. The risk of breast cancer is equal to that in non-users after 5 years off HRT.
    E. Women taking sequential HRT for more than 1 year are considered at higher risk of developing endometrial cancer.

97. The following **three** drugs are recommended for the management of mild benign prostatic hypertrophy:

    A. Cyproterone acetate
    B. Finasteride
    C. Indoramin
    D. Terazosin
    E. Tolterodine tartrate

98–102. Groin lumps

    A. Direct inguinal hernia
    B. Femoral hernia
    C. Incarcerated hernia
    D. Indirect inguinal hernia
    E. Psoas abscess
    F. Saphena varix

For each of the clinical examination findings below select the **single** most likely diagnosis from the above list of options:

98. A small lump is palpated in the groin medially. It transmits a cough impulse. It disappears when the patient lies down.

99. A lump arising in the superficial inguinal canal is felt on your fingertip when the patient coughs.

100. A lump arising in the superficial inguinal canal is felt against the pulp of your finger when the patient coughs.

101. A fluctuant mass is palpated in the groin of an indigent. He also c/o back pain and is found to have a swinging pyrexia.

102. A 35-year-old woman presents with a mass above the inguinal ligament pointing downwards to the thigh. The lump is felt below and lateral to the pubic tubercle.

103–106. Immunological investigations

    A. Anti-mitochondrial antibody
    B. Anti-neutrophil cytoplasmic antibody
    C. Antibody against double-stranded DNA
    D. Anti-phospholipid antibody
    E. Antibody to reticulin
    F. Rheumatoid factor
    G. Thyroid antibodies

For each of the patients below select from the list of options above the **single** most discriminating investigation:

103. A 40-year-old woman presents with a photosensitive malar rash over both cheeks and the bridge of her nose, and chronic musculoskeletal pain.

104. A 30-year-old woman presents with 3 recurrent miscarriages. She also suffers from chronic migraines.

105. A 40-year-old woman presents with itching, jaundice and upper GI bleed.

106. A 60-year-old man presents with recurrent epistaxis, hypertension and microscopic haematuria.

107–112. Evidence-based treatment of metastatic breast carcinoma

A. Aminoglutethimide
B. High-dose chemotherapy
C. Megestrol
D. Paclitaxel
E. Radiotherapy
F. Standard-dose chemotherapy
G. Stilboestrol
H. Tamoxifen
I. Trilostane

For each of the conditions below, select the **single** most appropriate evidence-based treatment from the above list of options:

107. First-line therapy for estrogen receptor-positive widespread carcinoma

108. Bony metastases

109. For relapse on tamoxifen

110. Does not improve survival in patients who have undergone standard-dose chemotherapy

111. Is recommended by NICE for the treatment of advanced breast cancer where initial cytotoxic chemotherapy has failed or is inappropriate

112. Is tolerated with a PPI and corticosteroids

113. Which of the following methods may be used for management of scars?

A. Acrylic casts
B. Intralesional corticosteroid injection
C. Laser therapy
D. Silicon sheeting
E. Static splints

114–116. Red book

    A. Basic practice
    B. Capitation
    C. Cost
    D. Initial practice
    E. Notional

For each of the numbered gaps select the **single** word from the above list of options that best completes the sentence. Each option may be used once, more than once, or not at all.

A practitioner building a new separate purpose-built premises may be reimbursed a (114) _____ rent. A pre-agreed percentage of the total cost of the building is reimbursed to the practitioner each year. Owner-occupiers are paid (115) _____ rent allowance for allowing use of their private building for NHS purposes. The rent payment is based on the current market rent value assessed by the district valuer. New partners are expected to buy into the practice if the allowance is based on (116) ____ rent.

117. According to Groves' classification, the different types of heart-sink patients are:

    A. Aggressive manipulators
    B. Entitled demanders
    C. Dependent clingers
    D. Manipulative help-rejectors
    E. Self-destructive deniers

118. Exceptions to generic prescribing include:

    A. Anticonvulsants
    B. Ciclosporin
    C. Diltiazem
    D. Nifedipine
    E. Theophylline

119. Deaths that need to be reported to the coroner include: (*OHGP*)

    A. Death through neglect
    B. Death due to industrial disease
    C. Deceased not attended by a doctor in their last illness
    D. Deceased not seen by the doctor completing the death certificate after death
    E. Infant deaths

120. Identify from the following list the **three** substances that have been shown to cause occupational asthma:

A. Flour
B. Glutaraldehyde
C. Isocyanate
D. Lead
E. Nickel

121–125. Childhood rashes

A. Chickenpox
B. Erythema multiforme
C. Erythema nodosum
D. Kawasaki disease
E. Hand-foot-and-mouth disease
F. Herpes simplex
G. Measles
H. Molluscum contagiosum
I. Scarlet fever

For each of the patients below select from the list of options above the **single** most likely diagnosis:

121. A 10-year-old boy presents with three pale umbilicated papules on his neck. He enjoys swimming at school.

122. A 3-year-old girl presents with painful mouth ulcers and red spots on her palms. She is not unwell.

123. A 15-year-old girl presents with crops of pale erythematous-violaceous macules surrounded by concentric rings on her palms. She had taken a course of penicillin.

124. A 2-year-old boy presents with high fever and a morbilliform rash that started over his forehead and cheeks and has now spread to his trunk and limbs. He has a hoarse cough and his mouth is painful and red.

125. A 7-year-old boy presents with a sore throat and a truncal rash of pink coalescent rings. He has a strawberry tongue.

126. Which **four** of the following are examples of longitudinal studies?

    A. Case–control studies
    B. Cohort studies
    C. Prevalence studies
    D. Prospective studies
    E. Retrospective studies

127. The **four** factors influencing predicted normal lung function values include:

    A. Age
    B. Ethnic origin
    C. Height
    D. Sex
    E. Weight

128. The **single** best treatment for scalp ringworm in children is:

    A. Clotrimazole cream
    B. Ketoconazole shampoo
    C. Oral griseofulvin
    D. Oral itraconazole
    E. Terbinafine cream

129. The following are recognized treatments for cradle cap:

    A. Arachis oil
    B. Betadine shampoo
    C. Capasal shampoo
    D. Cocois scalp ointment
    E. Olive oil

130. Which **two** statements regarding treatment for migraines are true?

    A. Beta-blockers may be used for migraine prophylaxis.
    B. Ergot alkaloids may be prescribed prophylactically.
    C. Ismethoptene mucate in combination with paracetamol is licensed for the treatment of migraines.
    D. Pizotifen may be used for treatment of acute attacks.
    E. $5HT_1$ antagonists are useful in the treatment of acute attacks.

131–141. Evidence-based management of anaemia

A. Anaemia of chronic disease
B. Assess iron status
C. Blood film
D. B_{12}
E. Beta- or alpha-thalassaemia trait
F. DAT reticulocyte count
G. ESR
H. Hb electrophoresis
I. History of diet, drugs and alcohol
J. Iron deficiency anaemia
K. LFTs

For each of the numbered gaps, choose **one** word from the above list:

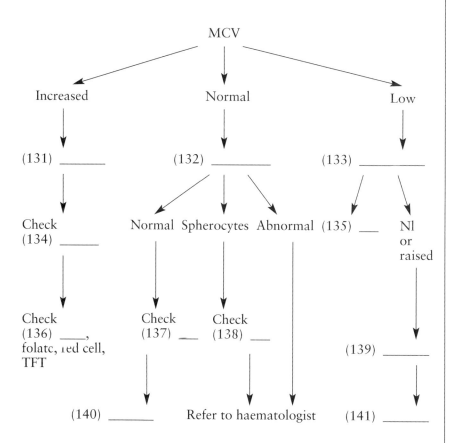

142. A 70-year-old woman presents with swollen lower legs. She is on 5 mg of felodipine for hypertension and indomethacin for rheumatic disease. Her BP is currently 140/70. The **single** most appropriate step is:

A. Add a loop diuretic
B. Add a thiazide diuretic
C. Change felodipine to an ACE inhibitor
D. Change indomethacin to a COX-2 inhibitor
E. Prescribe elastic stockings

143. A 30-year-old woman complains of headaches, feeling TAT and disoriented. She reports that she moved into a council flat in November. The flat is damp with visible mould. She also suffers from asthma and is on Dianette for contraception. The **single** most appropriate management would be:

A. Advise testing for carbon monoxide poisoning.
B. Arrange patch testing for mould sensitization.
C. Change Dianette to POP.
D. Increase inhalers since patient is allergic to mould.
E. Prescribe antidepressant.

144–150. Welfare benefits

Match the following allowances with their correct descriptions:

A. Attendance allowance
B. Disabled concessions
C. Disability living allowance
D. Disability working allowance
E. Incapacity benefits
F. Income support
G. Invalid care allowance
H. Severe disability allowance
I. Social fund benefits
J. Unemployment benefit

144. A tax-free, non-means-tested allowance for a person over the age of 65 with a severe physical or mental disability requiring care during the day or day and night.

145. An allowance for a person aged between 18 and 65 with > or equal to 80% disability who is unable to work for 28 weeks. NI contributions are not mandatory.

146. A tax-free but income-related and means-tested allowance for a person on low income who is older than 16 and works at least 16 hours a week and is receiving one of the disability allowances.

147. This is paid at 3 different rates (short-term at lower rate, short-term at higher rate and long-term after 1 year) to a person unfit for work on medical grounds for > 28 weeks and who has paid NI contributions.

148. This includes assistance with travel fares, council tax relief, exemption from road tax, free dental care, free glasses and free prescriptions and social services assistance.

149. This will pay for cold weather, funeral and maternity expenses, i.e. exceptional expenses.

150. This is paid to a person between the ages of 5 and 65 who requires care and is unable to walk for 3 months.

151. The **single** drug of choice for neuropathic pain is: (*BMJ Clinical Evidence*)

    A. Amitriptyline
    B. Capsaicin
    C. Carbamazepine
    D. Gabapentin
    E. Tramadol

152. A 40-year-old woman presents with a swollen left wrist. She works as a hotel maid. On examination there is swelling over the styloid process of the radius with pain on forced flexion and adduction of the thumb. The **single** most likely diagnosis is:

    A. Carpal tunnel syndrome
    B. De Quervain's disease
    C. Dupuytren's contracture
    D. Scaphoid fracture
    E. Trigger thumb

153. Select **two** correct statements regarding the 2003 NICE guidelines for the treatment of influenza A or B:

    A. Amantadine may be used for both prophylaxis and treatment of influenza in the same household.
    B. Oseltamivir is recommended for the treatment of influenza A or B in at-risk patients who can start on treatment within 48 hours of symptom onset.
    C. Patients with diabetes are included in the at-risk patient group for influenza.
    D. Zanamivir is recommended for patients over the age of 60 who can start on treatment within 72 hours of symptom onset.
    E. Zanamivir may be used for the treatment of influenza in healthy adults.

154. Select **two** correct statements regarding smallpox:

    A. In light of the threat of pox virus being used as a terrorist weapon, mass immunization is needed.
    B. The smallpox virus was certified by the World Health Organization as eradicated in 1979.
    C. In the event of an outbreak, the Department of Health plans to contain and ring-vaccinate, isolating and vaccinating contacts.
    D. According to the DoH, all healthcare personnel across the UK are being offered vaccination.
    E. Variola virus is an RNA virus.

155–159. Asylum or refugee status definitions

    A. Asylum seeker
    B. Exceptional leave to enter
    C. Exceptional leave to remain
    D. Family reunion
    E. Refugee status
    F. Refusal

    Match the following definitions with the terms above:

155. One spouse and children of that marriage under the age of 18 are given indefinite leave to remain.

156. The Home Office accepts there are strong reasons why the person should not return to their country of origin.

157. A person who has submitted an application for protection under the 1951 Geneva Convention and is waiting for their claim to be settled by the Home Office.

158. A person who is granted indefinite leave to remain – permanent residence in the UK – and is eligible for family reunion.

159. A discretionary status for varying periods depending on age and other circumstances. The person is expected to return if the situation in the country of origin improves.

160. Select **two** correct statements regarding low back pain:

    A. Lumbar disc prolapse most commonly affects the 30- to 40-year-old age group.
    B. Lumbar spine x-ray is often useful in the acute setting.
    C. Patients with concomitant urinary retention should be referred urgently for spinal decompression.
    D. Surgical discectomy for prolapsed lumbar disc is much more effective than chymopapain injections.
    E. Two weeks' bedrest is a first-line treatment option.

161. Select **two** correct statements regarding MMR vaccination:

    A. Children with leukaemia are at high risk and should be offered the MMR vaccine.
    B. The MMR vaccine contains live, attenuated viruses.
    C. The MMR vaccine is associated with autistic enterocolitis.
    D. The MMR vaccine is not safe in children who have had an anaphylactic reaction to eggs.
    E. The UK recommends two doses of MMR in childhood.

162. Select **two** correct statements regarding methotrexate:

    A. Any profound drop in white cell or platelet count calls for immediate reduction of methotrexate dose.
    B. Folinic acid is used to counteract the folate-agonist action of methotrexate and is given 24 hours prior to methotrexate.
    C. It is usually prescribed once weekly at a starting dose of 7.5 mg.
    D. It may induce pneumonitis.
    E. Patients require weekly full blood count and renal and liver function tests while on methotrexate.

163. Select **two** correct statements regarding Parkinson's disease:

   A. Antimuscarinic drugs improve tardive dyskinesia.
   B. Levodopa in combination with dopa-decarboxylase inhibitor is the treatment of choice.
   C. Non-coffee drinkers have a 30% reduction in risk compared with coffee drinkers.
   D. Non-smokers have a 60% reduction in risk of Parkinson's disease compared with cigarette smokers.
   E. Parkinson's is associated with a 4–6 Hz tremor, most marked at rest.

164. The following steps should be taken in the management of peripheral artery disease in primary care **except**:

   A. All patients should be on a statin to achieve a 25% reduction in cholesterol.
   B. Consider ACE inhibitors in all patients, even if normotensive.
   C. Prescribe aspirin 75 mg daily.
   D. Prescribe cilostazol for the first 3–6 months.
   E. Screen for type 2 diabetes.

165. Select **two** correct statements regarding plantar fasciitis:

   A. A bony spur projecting forwards from the undersurface of the calcaneal tuberosity is often seen on x-ray.
   B. Pain may be elicited on palpation 4 cm anterior to the heel.
   C. Patients should be referred to an orthopaedic outpatient clinic.
   D. Steroid injections are the mainstay of treatment.
   E. Stretching exercises to the Achilles tendon may be helpful.

166–173. Match the following studies with their correct descriptions:

   A. ASCOT
   B. CAPRIE
   C. CARE
   D. CURE
   E. DASH
   F. HOT
   G. ISIS-2
   H. MRFIT
   I. SHEP
   J. UKPDS

166. This trial showed that patients in the atenolol and bendrofluazide arm were more likely to develop diabetes than in the perindopril and amlodipine arm.

167. This trial showed that increasing blood pressure increases the relative risk of coronary heart disease, stroke and end-stage renal disease.

168. This trial showed that a diet rich in fruit, vegetables, low in fat and with reduced saturated and total fat, can substantially reduce blood pressure.

169. This trial showed that low-dose diuretic-based treatment is effective in preventing major CVD events, cardiac and cerebral, in both type 2 diabetes and non-diabetic older patients with ischaemic heart disease.

170. This trial showed that aspirin significantly reduced major CV events with the greatest benefit seen in all myocardial infarctions.

171. This trial showed that aggressive control of hypertension in diabetics led to a decrease in cardiovascular events.

172. This study showed that clopidogrel is as effective as aspirin in decreasing the risk of CV events.

173. This study showed that clopidogrel taken with aspirin for 6 months increases the anti-thrombotic effect of aspirin. However, the risk of bleeding is also increased.

174–177. Match the following terms with their correct definitions:
- A. Absolute risk
- B. Negative predictive value
- C. Positive predictive value
- D. Relative risk
- E. Sensitivity
- F. Specificity

174. The proportion of true positives correctly identified by the test.

175. The proportion of patients with a positive test who have been correctly identified as having the disease.

176. The ratio of disease incidence in the exposed versus the non-exposed group.

177. The proportion of true negatives correctly identified by the test.

178–181. Match the following studies with the most appropriate study design:

A. Case–control study
B. Cohort study
C. Cross-sectional study
D. Meta-analysis (Forest plot)
E. Randomized controlled study

178. A comparison of case fatalities in patients with diabetes versus those without, following an acute myocardial infarction.

179. A study to determine the percentage of babies born to mothers treated with thalidomide who developed limb hypoplasia.

180. A survey of 5 GP practices' anti-viral prescribing habits.

181. A comparison of trials looking at the risk of DVT with third-generation combined oral contraceptives.

182–184. Peripheral neuropathy (OHCM)

A. Charcot–Marie–Tooth disease
B. Chronic symmetrical peripheral neuropathy
C. Diabetic neuropathy
D. Guillain–Barré syndrome
E. Multiple compression palsy
F. Multiple sclerosis
G. Systematic vasculitis

For each of the patients below select the **single** most likely diagnosis from the above list of options. Each option may be used once, more than once, or not at all.

182. A 30-year-old man presents with distal paraesthesiae and distal or proximal weakness occurring 1–2 weeks after a GI infection. The reflexes are present initially but become absent within 1 hour. He soon loses the ability to walk and develops facial and bulbar weakness.

183. A 70-year-old woman with rheumatoid arthritis presents with rapid onset of multiple mononeuropathy.

184. A patient on cisplatin for metastatic seminoma presents with months of ataxia. He states that his gait is worse in the dark. No other members of his family have similar symptoms, claw toes or pes cavus. On examination the neuropathy is confirmed as sensory and subacute.

185–192. Evidence-based advances in breast cancer

    A. Anastrozole (third-line aromatase inhibitors)
    B. Axillary dissection
    C. Fulvestrant (selective oestrogen receptor downregulators)
    D. Prophylactic mastectomy
    E. Prophylactic oophorectomy
    F. Sentinel node biopsy
    G. Surveillance
    H. Tamoxifen

For each of the numbered gaps, choose one **single** option from the list above that best completes the sentence. Each option may be used once, more than once, or not at all.

Hartmann et al reviewed over 6000 women with a family history of breast cancer who underwent (185)_____ and determined that reduction in death from breast cancer ranged from 81% to 94%. (186)_____ reduces the risk of breast cancer by approximately 50% in *BRCA1* carriers. (187)_____ has fewer complications than (188) _____ and is contraindicated in cases of pregnancy, multi-centric carcinoma and suspicious palpable axillary adenopathy. (189) _____ was until recently the standard first-line treatment for oestrogen receptor-positive metastatic cancer. Evidence-based medicine now suggests (190) _____ as first-line treatment in premenopausal women. In a North American trial of 400 postmenopausal women with metastatic disease recurring or progressing on tamoxifen, (191) _____ rather than (192) _____was found to increase time to disease progression, increase rate of clinical benefit and lengthen duration of response.

193–197. Evidence-based management of lower urinary tract symptoms in men

A. Alpha-blockers
B. Antimuscarinic drugs
C. 5-α reductase inhibitors
D. Prostatectomy
E. Reduce fluid intake in the evening and avoid caffeine
F. Referral for specialist assessment
G. *Serenoa repens*
H. TURP

For each of the numbered gaps, choose **one** option from the above list that best completes the sentence. Each option may be used once, more than once, or not at all.

Men with uncomplicated lower urinary tract symptoms arising from benign enlargement of the prostate should be offered (193) _____ initially. If troublesome symptoms persist, (194) _____ should be offered for 2–4 weeks. If men do not respond, cannot tolerate the side effects or the prostate is estimated to be greater than 40 ml, (195) _____ should be offered. Evidence-based medicine has shown that (196) _____ improved overall self-rated urinary symptoms from baseline compared with placebo but long-term safety has not been addressed. Men with visible haematuria, dysuria, renal failure or urinary retention should be offered (197) _____.

198. Evidence-based medicine suggests that injectable adrenaline with oral antihistamine should be prescribed for any child who has had an allergic reaction with (select **three** correct answers):

A. A history of diabetes mellitus
B. A history of eczema
C. Mild respiratory symptoms
D. Occurrence on exposure to only a trace amount of allergen
E. Occurrence in a child who has asthma that requires regular inhaled corticosteroids

199. A 2-year-old girl presents with fever of 5 days, swollen hands and feet with peeling of the fingers and toes, strawberry tongue, cracked lips, non-tender cervical lymphadenopathy and a polymorphous truncal rash. Select the **two** best forms of treatment for this girl:

A. Acyclovir suspension
B. Aspirin
C. Calpol
D. IV benzylpenicillin
E. IV immunoglobulin

200. Urgent referrals to secondary care for depression should be made in which **four** of the following cases:

A. Child sexual abuse survivors
B. Depression in association with epilepsy
C. Depression with hallucinations
D. Elderly patients over the age of 65 with a first episode of depression
E. Expressed suicidal intent
F. Personality disorder
G. Postnatal depression
H. Severe retarded depression

Applied Knowledge Test Module Paper Two: Answers

1. D

2. B

3. E

4. E

5. CF

6. BCE

7. A.   Both alendronic acid and risedronate (both bisphosphonates) are available as once-weekly preparations, which is more amenable for patients who dislike daily tablets. The classic Dowager's Hump is pathognomonic for severe osteoporosis without imaging. A lateral back x-ray should be obtained if osteoporosis is suspected and confirmed by DEXA scan. A value > −2.5 standard deviations below the young adult female value is the WHO definition for osteoporosis. It is indefensible in a court of law if you do not put your patient on osteoporosis prophylaxis if you prescribe long-term corticosteroids. Recent evidence shows that repeated short courses of steroids may be more detrimental than long-term regular steroids! HRT is no longer recommended as prophylaxis against osteoporosis and should only be prescribed for 2–3 years maximum, for relief of troublesome menopausal symptoms.

8. ABDE.   Caution should be used in patients with DM.

9. BDE.   Anthrax has an incubation period of 1–7 days. It is a Gram-positive rod diagnosed in cultures from skin or nasal swabs or blood cultures. Three forms of disease include cutaneous (95%), pulmonary and ingestion. Cutaneous anthrax results in a black eschar (malignant pustule) 4–9 days after exposure. Oedema, fever and hepatosplenomegaly may also be present. This form responds to oral ciprofloxacin. Only those directly exposed to spores should be given 60 days of oral ciprofloxacin 500 mg bd. CXR findings with pulmonary anthrax include widened mediastinum, lymphadenopathy and haemorrhagic mediastinitis. These findings can also occur with tuberculosis. The prognosis is poor.

10. ABCDE. Other notifiable diseases include anthrax, diphtheria, dysentery, Ebola virus, encephalitis, leprosy, leptospirosis, malaria, meningitis, meningococcal sepsis, mumps, ophthlamia neonatorum, plague, poliomyelitis, rabies, relapsing fever, rubella, tetanus, tuberculosis, typhus, viral haemorrhagic fevers (including Lassa fever), whooping cough and yellow fever.

11. A. Acute otitis media in a child < 2 years of age should be treated with antibiotics within 48 hours of onset of signs and symptoms of middle ear inflammation, especially with a T 39°C or greater. Observation is recommended for children over 6 months with an uncertain diagnosis, mild otalgia and T < 39°C. In children aged 2 years and older, antibiotics are only indicated in severe illness (moderate to severe otalgia or high fever with a certain diagnosis of otitis media).

12. ABCE. The British Heart Foundation published a fact-file sheet on CHD and air travel in December 2002. At 5,000 feet, due to the barometric pressure, PaO_2 on air is only 75 mmHg. At 8,000 feet, this figure is only 65 mmHg. The oxygen dissociation curve of normal haemoglobin allows for 90% saturation of haemoglobin at cabin altitudes but for patients with CHD where tissue perfusion is inadequate, this poses a problem. More information can be obtained from www.bhf.org.uk/factfiles.

13. D. It is imperative to refer a patient who has suffered a TIA to the rapid access TIA clinic within 1 week of the event to prevent high risk of subsequent full stroke.

14. CDE. In 2000, the RCP published evidence-based guidelines for the management of stroke. Aspirin should only be started after a CT scan of the head has excluded haemorrhage. Aspirin is indicated for ischaemic stroke. Dipyridamole is offered to patients already on aspirin. Thrombolysis is not routinely offered in the UK, unlike the US. Heparin prophylaxis is also indicated for prior thromboembolism. Heparin is also offered to patients with carotid artery dissection. Blood pressure is often high after a stroke and is only treated if it persists. About 75% survive an acute stroke and progress to rehab. Secondary prevention includes smoking cessation, reduction in alcohol and salt intake, mini-dose aspirin and statins if the patient is < 75 with evidence of carotid atheroma or h/o CHD. Patients with carotid artery stenosis or occlusion identified by carotid duplex studies may be offered endarterectomy.

15. A

16. D

17. C.   The Simvastatin Survival Study was the first trial of LDL-cholesterol lowering with statins for secondary prevention of CHD.

18. E

19. B.   Cholesterol and Recurrent Events (CARE).

20. ABCDE.   The British Renal Association recommends referral if the serum creatinine is > 150 µmol/L. Renal function should be monitored in patients on ACE inhibitors or angiotensin receptor II inhibitors to exclude renal artery stenosis. Many patients with occult atheromatous renal artery disease may end up with renal failure requiring dialysis.

21. ABD.   Sibutramine requires close monitoring of BP. Orlistat is associated with GI side effects.

22. E

23. A

24. C

25. B

26. F

27. G

28. B

29. E

30. D

31. C

32. A. Actual ECGs are popular in the new MCQ paper. Make sure you can differentiate between these three conditions on ECG.

33. C

34. B

35. ABDE. To reduce pressure on echocardiography services, NICE has implemented guidelines regarding NT-proBNP blood tests for heart failure. ACE inhibitors (ie enalapril) and not angiotensin receptor blockers (ARBs) are recommended as first-line therapy for CHF. Renal function must be monitored at the start of treatment and 2–3 weeks following when initiating ACE inhibitor therapy. Loop diuretics are also recommended as first-line therapy. ValHeFT (Valsartan in Heart Failure Trial) showed that ARBs may have a role in CHF in patients who are intolerant to ACE inhibitors and beta-blockers. Beta-blockers show their effect with chronic use and patients should be encouraged to persist with therapy. Use a lower dose in the elderly.

36. A. There is limited evidence that the cessation of cow's milk reduces baby colic, but this is a popular MRCGP question.

37. E

38. B. This woman has iron-deficiency anaemia secondary to menorrhagia from fibroids.

39. C. This woman may have ITP (idiopathic thrombocytopaenic purpura).

40. B. This man may have haemochromatosis, which is often asymptomatic. Ferritin will be raised and LFTs deranged.

41. C. This boy may have Henoch–Schönlein purpura. The platelet count will be normal as the defect is with the vasculature.

42. D. This elderly man may have multiple myeloma diagnosed by monoclonal globulin spike on serum electrophoresis, plasmacytoma on tissue biopsy or bone marrow plasmacytosis with > 30% plasma cells.

43. ABCDE. NICE guidelines October 2002 now advocate that type 2 diabetic patients also be tested annually for microalbuminuria and if present with a BP > 140/80, antihypertensive medication should be commenced. Statins and fibrates should be used to decrease total cholesterol and triglycerides to below 5.0 mmol/L and 3.0 mmol/L, respectively.

44. A. Dietary advice should always be offered with advice on lifestyle changes. It is important to assess CHD risk, as this will influence management. CHD risk factors include FHx of IHD, smoking, hypertension, diabetes, cerebrovascular or peripheral vascular disease or severe obesity. The British Hyperlipidaemia Association advocates a total cholesterol below 5 mmol/L and TG below 2.3 mmol/L. This patient's fasting lipid results are borderline. Referral to specialist lipid clinics is advised if the total cholesterol level is > 7.8 mmol/L or the triglycerides are > 4.5 mmol/L (risk of acute pancreatitis).

45. A. An FSH level > 30 IU/L with amenorrhoea is diagnostic of the menopause. HRT is now advocated for 2–3 years only and only for relief of distressing menopausal symptoms. HRT does not offer protection against osteoporosis or heart disease as has been suggested in the past.

46. ABCDE. Other risk groups for osteroporosis include patients with thoracic kyphosis, primary hypogonadism, previous fragility fracture, radiographic evidence of osteopenia, and chronic disorders associated with osteoporosis.

47. A. In children < 10 years of age, only 10% with glandular fever will have a positive monospot test. Also antibodies in glandular fever are transient and peak during the first 2 weeks after clinical onset. So adults may not develop a positive monospot test until a week later. If EBV is strongly suspected in a patient with a negative monospot test, immunofluorescence test is suggested for EBV-specific IgM or EBV serology for anti-EBNA1 IgG.

48. E. Rhinolast spray is useful for children aged 2–12 who suffer from allergic rhinitis. Senile watery rhinorrhoea is a non-allergic form of rhinitis.

49. E. Again this spray is for non-allergic rhinitis. Patients with nasal polyps should be commenced on a 2–3-month course of Betnesol drops. Larger polyps warrant a short course of corticosteroids and referral to ENT for a preop CT scan of the sinuses.

50. ABCDE.   According to the British Heart Foundation's Factfile sheet 01/2003 on pulmonary hypertension, severe symptomatic pulmonary hypertension warrants treatment in its own right. Bosentan is the newest licensed treatment for PPH. Sildenafil (Viagra) is under investigation as a potential form of treatment! There are 8 National Specialist Centres in the UK for the management of pulmonary hypertension.

51. D.   SSRIs can be used as first-line therapy although they may be slow to act. TCAs are often used for depression in the elderly but have numerous side effects – dry mouth, constipation, night sweats, drowsiness, dizziness, vivid dreams and fine tremor. Patients with cardiac arrhythmias on TCAs or with poorly controlled epilepsy should be offered SSRIs. A favourite trick is for the examiners to ask you for the second-line drug treatment. So read the question carefully.

52. C.   Olanzapine is an atypical antipsychotic without the extrapyramidal side effects of the older dopamine-blocking drugs. Clozapine is reserved for treatment of refractory schizophrenia and should only be administered in hospital. Piportal depot injections are reserved for patients who are unreliable with oral therapy.

53. D.   Acute pyelonephritis is associated with pyuria, >100,000 *E. coli*.

54. C.   Transitional cell carcinoma of the bladder is associated with microscopic haematuria and a sterile pyuria.

55. E.   Diabetes insipidus is associated with low urine osmolality.

56. A.   Renal calculus presents with severe colic and gross haematuria. It may be associated with a UTI.

57. B.   Renal tuberculosis presents with dysuria, haematuria and sterile pyuria.

58. AC.   It is now recommended **not** to bathe prior to treatment. Transmission is through direct skin contact and symptoms result from an immune reaction to the mites' saliva and faeces.

59. AE. Clothing lice are not treated with insecticides. They live in clothing and will die if clothing is not worn for 3 days or more. However, they can survive in clothes worn for long periods of time. Treatment is a shower or bath and washing infested clothing and bedding in hot water > 60°C.

60. B. The Mirena coil (levonorgestrel-releasing IUS) has an added benefit of reducing menstrual flow and dysmenorrhoea. Its contraceptive effect is by inducing endometrial atrophy and a hostile cervical mucus.

61. C. This woman may have emergency contraception in the form of Levonelle-2 up to 72 hours after UPSI. After that, the copper coil is recommended for emergency contraception for UPSI up to 5 days prior.

62. H

63. F. The COC can also be offered to patients with endometriosis (tricycling) to control symptoms.

64. D. This form of contraception is very popular in young women who can be forgetful and miss pills. Diarrhoea, vomiting and antibiotics all affect the efficacy of the pill. The POP, if offered, must be taken within the same 3-hour window period each day!

65. I. This woman can be offered either LAM for the first 6 months postpartum as long as she is amenorrhoeic and is fully breastfeeding or she can be offered Depo-Provera or POP.

66. C

67. G

68. F. Any NSAIDs (diclofenac, indomethacin or naproxen) may be prescribed. In my experience, patients prefer naproxen. IM Depo-Medrone works fast on inflammation but is not readily available to GPs. Allopurinol must never be commenced during an acute attack or it will make matters much worse. Do not prescribe colchicine first-line or you will be adding diarrhoea and vomiting to the patient's existing pain.

69. E. COX-2 inhibitors are contraindicated in patients with heart failure. Methotrexate should be prescribed at a starting dose of 7.5 mg once weekly with 5 mg of folic acid weekly for potential mucosal or GI side effects. MTX requires regular FBC, U/E and LFTs.

70. D

71. C. According to the National Disease Surveillance Centre, vomit should be cleaned with a dilute bleach solution (0.1% hypochlorite) to ensure destruction of the Norwalk-like virus (NLV) which is transmitted through the vomit of an infected individual. Sodium perborate is an antiseptic mouthwash and is similar to hydrogen peroxide and chlorhexidine.

72. ABCDE. Antiphospholipid syndrome occurs with SLE and requires close supervision during pregnancy. Mothers are commenced on aspirin and may require S/C heparin or warfarin. The baby is at risk of placental insufficiency, IUGR, and fetal death.

73. ABCDEF. An easy mnemonic to remember the drugs that cause gout is CANT LEAP (ciclosporin, alcohol, nicotinic acid, thiazides, loop diuretics, ethambutol, aspirin and pyrazinamide). Consequently, one of the risks of anti-tuberculosis therapy is gout!

74. F

75. E. This woman may have primary biliary cirrhosis, a slow, chronic liver disease.

76. B. This man most likely has haemochromatosis. The definitive investigation is liver biopsy. Diabetes should be excluded in this man.

77. A. This man most likely has a stone in the common bile duct.

78. D. This farmer may have extrinsic allergic alveolitis. Treatment is removal of allergen, oxygen, IV hydrocortisone and oral prednisolone.

79. E. This man is presenting with signs of heart failure and would benefit from an ACE inhibitor.

80. F. This man would benefit from a trial of salbutamol.

81. D. This man may have sarcoidosis.

82. C. Tickly cough is a side effect of ACE inhibitors, in which case angiotensin II-receptor antagonists may be substituted.

83. B. This man will most likely have an atypical pneumonia. If the infection does not clear, he may need a chest and hand x-ray to exclude tuberculosis.

84. A. Age is no bar to holding a licencse. A 3-year licence is issued as long as the patient at age 70 confirms with the DVLA that no medical disability is present.

85. F. Persistent BP of 180/100 or greater disqualifies a group 2 entitlement driver.

86. G. The DVLA must be notified and driving cease if cerebral metastases are present.

87. C. If the operation required was a craniotomy, the patient would be barred for 12 months.

88. A. Colour blindness is no bar to driving.

89. D. A drug misuser is automatically disqualified for a minimum of 12 months. However with close supervision on a methadone programme, he may reapply subject to annual medical review and favourable assessment.

90. A. A single confirmed episode of transient global amnesia is no bar to group 2 entitlement. However if two or more episodes occurred, driving would be banned until investigated further.

91. B. Corticosteroids induce remission in > 90% of children.

92. E.   There is a poor response to corticosteroids (10–30%). Cyclophosphamide or ciclosporin may be used.

93. G.   Other associations include malignancy, drugs, autoimmune conditions and infections. Treatment involves corticosteroids and chlorambucil (Ponticelli regimen).

94. I.   Treatment involves high-dose corticosteroids, cyclophosphamide $\pm$ plasma exchange or renal transplant. Prognosis is poor if the initial serum creatinine level is > 600 µmol/L.

95. F.   There is no treatment and half will progress to end-stage renal failure.

96. ABD.   HRT is associated with increased risk of endometrial cancer after 5 years of sequential use. Raloxifene (the first SERM) is not useful for the management of menopausal symptoms and is associated with a 2–3-fold increase in VTE but is used to treat osteoporosis. In a RCT in 7705 osteoporotic women treated with raloxifene, the BMD was higher and the relative risk of vertebral fracture (0.5–0.7) was lower than in the placebo-arm.

97. BCD.   Cyproterone acetate is an anti-androgen used in the treatment of severe hypersexuality. Tolterodine is an antimuscarinic drug used to treat urinary frequency. Finasteride is an anti-androgen (5α-reductase inhibitor) that acts slowly on the size of the prostate and reduces risk of retention. Patients must be warned to use a condom as it is secreted in the semen. Alpha-blockers are used in patients awaiting a TURP.

98. F.   Saphena varix may also be associated with a bluish tinge to the skin.

99. D

100. A

101. E.   This man may well have Pott's disease.

102. B

103. C. This woman may have SLE.

104. D

105. A. This woman may have primary biliary cirrhosis.

106. B. This man may have Wegener's granulomatosis.

107. H

108. E

109. F

110. B

111. D. Paclitaxel is a taxane and is the treatment of choice for ovarian cancer. Both paclitaxel and docetaxel are also used for the treatment of advanced or metastatic breast cancer as per NICE guidelines.

112. I. Trilostane has a minor role in post-menopausal breast cancer that has relapsed following oestrogen antagonist therapy. As it inhibits the synthesis of mineralocorticoids and glucocorticoids, concomitant corticosteroid replacement therapy is required.

113. ABCDE. Management of scars may be divided into leave alone, non-invasive and invasive methods. Invasive methods include surgical excision and resuture, resurfacing, peel, dermabrasion, reconstruction with skin grafts, laser therapy, cryotherapy, bleomycin and fluorouracil injections.

114. C

115. E

116. E

117. BCDE.   There are 4 types.

118. ABCDE.   Drugs with narrow therapeutic range or modified-release preparations with different bioavailability should not be prescribed generically.

119. ABCDE

120. ABC.   Nurses are exposed to glutaraldehyde when disinfecting endoscopes.

121. H

122. E

123. B

124. G

125. I

126. ABDE

127. ABCD

128. C.   Only oral griseofulvin is licensed in the UK to be used to treat tinea capitis in children. Anti-fungal creams do not penetrate the hair-shaft.

129. ACE.   Betadine shampoo and Cocois scalp ointment are not recommended in children under 2 and 6, respectively.

130. AC.   Serotonin agonists (ie sumatriptan, naratriptan and rizatriptan) are used for the treatment of acute attacks. Ergot alkaloids should never be used prophylactically; they are also associated with many side effects – GI upset and muscle cramps. Pizotifen is useful for the prevention of migraines.

131. I

132. C

133. B

134. K

135. J

136. D

137. G

138. F

139. H

140. A

141. E

142. C. Calcium channel blockers may be associated with gravitational oedema.

143. A. The flat may not have central heating and if the walls are mouldy then concern arises as to whether there is a gas leak from poor gas maintenance also. Carbon monoxide poisoning indoors increases during winter and the risk of dying is greater in the 2 million households that rely on solid fuel.

144. A

145. H

146. D

147. E

148. B

149. I

150. C

151. A. Starting dose of amitriptyline should be 10 mg nocte and increased slowly up to 75 mg if necessary. Carbamazepine and gabapentin are second-line drugs. Tramadol is used for nociceptive pain. Topical capsaicin has been used for neuropathic pain but some patients cannot tolerate the initial increase in pain.

152. B. Pain on forced flexion and adduction of the thumb is a positive Finckelstein's sign for De Quervain's tenosynovitis (stenosing tenovaginitis). The cause of the condition is unknown; however, wringing motions of the hands, e.g. drying out clothes, aggravate the condition. Treatment may involve steroid injection around the tendons or surgical decompression.

153. BC. Both oseltamivir and zanamivir have been approved by NICE in 2003 for the treatment of adults at risk of influenza A or B who can start on treatment within 48 hours of symptom onset. Oseltamivir is recommended for children who are at risk. At-risk categories include patients over the age of 65, patients with COPD or asthma, DM, significant CV disease (excluding hypertension), or those with immunosuppression).

154. BC. The DoH plans to offer vaccination to 350 key healthcare personnel across the UK (12 Smallpox Response Groups established around the UK) who would provide the first response in the event of a confirmed, suspected or threatened release of smallpox (a DNA pox virus).

155. D

156. B

157. A

158. E

159. C

160. CD.   Prolapsed lumbar disc is most common in the 20- to 30-year-old age group. The discs involved are L4/5 or L5/S1. 90% of patients are better within 6 weeks and 95% by 3 months. Gentle early mobilization and physiotherapy with analgesia is advocated. The Cochrane review from 2001 concluded that bed rest was not effective and may be deleterious.

161. BE

162. CD.   Methotrexate-induced pneumonitis is treated with corticosteroids. The Committee on Safety of Medicines has recommended a new warning label on methotrexate after numerous medication errors and overdosing. Methotrexate is usually given once weekly for the treatment of leukaemia, psoriasis and rheumatic disease. Folic acid is given once weekly after the dose of methotrexate to counteract the folate-antagonist effect of methotrexate. Blood tests are recommended before treatment commences and weekly until therapy stabilizes. Thereafter patients should be monitored every 2–3 months. Any drastic drop in white cell or platelet count calls for immediate withdrawal of methotrexate and administration of supportive therapy.

163. BE.   The first two options are reversed. Nicotine and caffeine have been proven to play a protective role in the development of Parkinson's disease. Antimuscarinics are used to reduce tremor and rigidity but can worsen tardive dyskinesia.

164. D.   Cilostazol is a useful adjunct in patients who have unacceptable symptoms despite 3–6 months of best medical treatment and has been shown to increase walking distance in patients with claudication.

165. BE

166. A

167. H

168. E

169. I

170. F

171. J

172. B

173. D

174. E.   As sensitivity has 'si' in the word, a useful tip is to associate this with the word sick. As specificity has 'fi' in the word, a useful tip is to associate this with the word fit.

175. C

176. D

177. F

178. A

179. A

180. C

181. D

182. D.   Guillain–Barré is an example of acute symmetrical peripheral neuropathy, which can be fatal. Patients may not have absent reflexes in the first few hours of the disease. Treatment with IV immunoglobulin expedites recovery and reduces disability.

183. G.   Multiple mononeuropathy in a patient with a connective tissue disorder is most likely due to vasculitis. Treatment is with steroids $\pm$ cyclophosphamide.

184. B. Cisplatin and an underlying neoplasm are both associated with chronic symmetrical peripheral neuropathy. Charcot–Marie–Tooth is autosomal dominant so cannot be included in the differential.

185. D

186. E

187. F

188. B

189. H

190. A

191. C

192. A

193. E

194. A

195. C

196. G. Herbal therapy is available from health shops and may offer mild-to-moderate improvements in uncomplicated symptoms.

197. F

198. CDE

199. BE. This patient has features of Kawasaki's disease. Young children suspected of having this disease should be referred urgently for prompt treatment to prevent coronary artery damage.

200. CEGH. All the other cases may be referred on a routine basis.

Applied Knowledge Test Module Paper Three: Questions

1–6. Evidence-based treatment of psoriasis

A. Acitretin
B. Betamethasone
C. Calcipotriol
D. Coal tar
E. Ciclosporin
F. Dithranol
G. Hydroxyurea
H. Methotrexate
I. PUVB
J. PUVA
K. Tazarotene

Match each following description with the respective drug above:

1. Contains polycyclic aromatic hydrocarbon – known carcinogens.

2. Is useful for acute, generalized pustular psoriasis, psoriatic arthritis, psoriatic erythroderma and for psoriasis not responsive to topical therapy alone.

3. Is contraindicated in pregnancy but is the oral retinoid treatment of choice.

4. Has side effects of hypertension and kidney damage.

5. Causes permanent staining of bedding and clothing.

6. Is a vitamin D analogue.

7–11. Diagnosis of facial rashes

   A. Atopic dermatitis
   B. Cellulitis
   C. Contact dermatitis
   D. Dermatomyositis
   E. Discoid lupus erythematosus
   F. Impetigo
   G. Perioral dermatitis
   H. Psoriasis
   I. Rosacea
   J. Seborrhoeic dermatitis

For each of the patients below, select the **single** most appropriate diagnosis from the above list of options. Each option may be used once, more than once, or not at all:

7. A 4-year-old girl presents with a superficial erythematous rash with a golden-coloured crust around her nose, cheeks and mouth. She is systemically well.

8. A 20-year-old woman presents with a burning, itchy rash around her mouth. The eruption spares the skin around the vermilion border of her lips.

9. A 4-month-old baby boy presents with an itchy red rash over his cheeks. His mother suffers from asthma.

10. A 40-year-old woman reports facial flushing. On examination she has erythema, papules, pustules and telangiectasia on the nose and cheeks. The facial flushing is made worse by alcohol and sun exposure.

11. A 20-year-old woman presents with several months of facial rash. It started out with polymorphic, red scaly plaques and progressed to follicular plugging, scarring and hypopigmentation. The rash is made worse by sun exposure.

12–24. New GMS contract

A. Actual
B. Additional
C. Essential
D. GP
E. Less
F. Local-enhanced
G. More
H. National-enhanced
I. Opt-in
J. Opt-out
K. Out-of-hours
L. PCT
M. PMS
N. Practice
O. Quality
P. Weighted

For each of the numbered gaps, choose **one** word from the above list that best completes the sentence. Each option may be used once, more than once, or not at all.

The new GMS contract is a (12) _____-based contract. It offers 4 types of services in the national menu. Normal services include (13) _____ and (14) _____. Supplementary services include (15) _____ and (16) _____. Rewards for (17) _____ is an (18) _____ service. Out-of-hours is an (19) _____ service. Every (20) _____ has to offer a national-enhanced service. Care for asylum seekers and the homeless are examples of (21) _____ service. Service to violent patients or to cover minor injuries are examples of (22) _____ service. Global sum calculation is based on number of (23) _____ patients list size. Therefore, a practice with a clean list based in a high inflation area will get (24) _____ money.

25–29. Evidence-based management of lower back pain

A. Advise bedrest and NSAIDs.
B. Arrange prompt investigation or referral within 4 weeks.
C. Assess for yellow flags.
D. Continue normal daily activities and prescribe paracetamol.
E. Emergency referral.
F. Specialist referral if no better in 4 weeks after conservative management.

For each of the clinical cases below, select the **single** best management option from the above list. Each option may be used once, more than once or not at all.

25. A 50-year-old man presents with lumbosacral pain without sciatica.

26. A 56-year-old man presents with thoracic back pain and weight loss. On examination he has structural deformity and widespread neurological symptoms.

27. A 30-year-old woman presents with buttock pain radiating down to her toes. SLR reproduces the pain.

28. A 60-year-old man presents with urinary incontinence, saddle anaesthesia and relenting back pain.

29. A 40-year-old man requests repeated med3 certs for low back pain.

30–36. Roles of committees

A. CHI
B. Clinical Governance
C. GMC
D. GPC (GMSC)
E. LMC
F. NCAA
G. NICE
H. PACT

Match the following roles with the correct respective committee from the above list.

30. It is the sole negotiating body with the Department of Health and is a standing committee of the BMA and represents all GPs in the UK.

31. It is a statutory body of locally elected GPs who meet monthly locally and annually at a national conference.

32. This analyses prescribing patterns and cost data for each practice and compares them with other practices in the area.

33. This committee oversees the quality of clinical governance and of services. It was established in April 2000 and reviews all types of organizations, e.g. GP practices, hospitals, PCTs, regarding their quality of services to patients.

34. This produces and disseminates clinical guidelines to promote cost-effective therapies and uniform clinical standards. It covers guidance on health technology, clinical management of specific conditions, and referral guidelines from primary to secondary care.

35. This is an initiative of the White Paper *The New NHS* and is a framework to improve patient care through high standards, personal and team development and cost-effective, evidence-based clinical practice.

36. This authority assesses a doctor's performance rapidly to avoid years of suspension during an enquiry.

37. A tympanic membrane with chalky-white patches is **best** associated with:

    A. Cholesteatoma
    B. Chronic serous otitis media
    C. Noise-induced hearing loss
    D. Otosclerosis
    E. Tympanosclerosis

38. Select **three** correct statements listed on a patient's steroid card:

    A. I am a patient on steroid treatment, which must not be stopped suddenly.
    B. If you come into contact with chickenpox, see your doctor urgently.
    C. For 1 year after you stop treatment, you must mention that you have taken steroids.
    D. If you have taken this medicine for more than 3 weeks but less than 6, you may stop treatment suddenly.
    E. If you have never had chickenpox, see your doctor for antibody testing.

39. Select the **single** best answer definition of the black triangle symbol in the *BNF*.

    A. Denotes those preparations that are considered by the Joint Formulary Committee to be less suitable for prescribing.
    B. Identifies newly licensed medicines that are monitored intensively by the MCA/CSM and requires all suspected reactions to be reported through the Yellow Card scheme.
    C. Identifies preparations that are not available for NHS prescription.
    D. Identifies prescription-only medicines.
    E. Requires handwritten requests on FP-10 prescriptions.

40. A 30-year-old woman requests a prescription for Dianette for con-traception. Select the **single** correct answer regarding this prescription:

   A. As Dianette is also used to treat acne, the patient will be charged private prices.
   B. Is contraindicated as a form of contraception in diabetic patients.
   C. The prescription must be handwritten.
   D. The prescription should contain the female sign.
   E. This pill comes in a 28-day pack.

41–45. Drug misuse

   A. Ask patient to produce urine specimen on premises for urine toxicology to confirm presence of opiates.
   B. Introduce mirtazapine and wean off diazepam.
   C. Prescribe and maintain on current dose of diazepam.
   D. Prescribe heroin.
   E. Prescribe methadone on handwritten FP10.
   F. Refer to dual team.
   G. Refer to in-patient detox centre.
   H. Refer to specialist GP in drug misuse or community drug team.

For each of the following patients below select the **single** most appropriate evidence-based management from the above list of options. Each option may be used once, more than once, or not at all.

41. A 40-year-old IVDA demands methadone as he wants to come off heroin. He states that he will steal if you do not prescribe methadone. (**Two** best answers)

42. A 30-year-old IVDA on methadone informs you that he has lost his prescription and has missed 3 days of methadone. He requests a repeat prescription. (**Two** best answers)

43. A 30-year-old man with a history of schizophrenia and heroin misuse presents for drug management.

44. A 50-year-old man requests Antabuse as he wishes to give up alcohol.

45. A 45-year-old woman requests a repeat prescription for diazepam. She has taken 2 mg diazepam nocte for the past year for anxiety and depression.

46. A court order for release of patient's medical records without a patient's written consent is called:

A. Order of determination
B. Order of disclosure
C. Order of discovery
D. Order of public interest
E. Order of release of medical records

47. A 22-year-old man develops asthma 2 years after starting work in a bakery. The **two** best tests to confirm flour allergy are:

A. Chest x-ray
B. Patch test
C. RAST
D. Serum IgE
E. Skin prick test

48. Extrinsic allergic alveolitis is a form of which type of hypersensitivity reaction:

A. I
B. II
C. III
D. IV
E. V

49. A 50-year-old woman with rheumatoid arthritis is unable to tolerate both sulfasalazine and methotrexate. She has been on indomethacin for the past 3 years. The **single** most appropriate alternative treatment is:

A. Ciclosporin
B. Leflunomide
C. Misoprostol
D. Naproxen
E. Rofecoxib

50–54. Foot pain

A. Arthritis of the subtalar joint
B. Freiberg's disease
C. Hallux rigidus
D. Kohler's disease
E. Metatarsalgia
F. Morton's metatarsalgia
G. Osteochondritis
H. Plantar fasciitis
I. Postcalcaneal bursitis
J. Stress fracture

For each of the patients below select the **single** most appropriate diagnosis from the above list of options. Each option may be used once, more than once or not at all.

50. A 4-year-old boy complains of painful foot and limps. On examination, pain is felt in the mid-tarsal area. X-ray confirms dense, deformed bone.

51. A 45-year-old woman presents with pain on the underside of the heel. She reports that it is worse first thing in the morning and eases with walking. Walking up stairs makes the pain worse.

52. A 27-year-old marathon runner presents with pain in the shaft of the 2nd metatarsal. X-ray is normal.

53. A 20-year-old airline stewardess complains of pain in the 3rd and 4th toes. Pain is elicited on compression of the affected web space.

54. An 11-year-old girl presents with forefoot pain. On x-ray the epiphysis of the 2nd metatarsal head is flattened, fragmented and granular.

55. Papillary thyroid cancer is most frequent in which **two** of the following decades:

A. 20s
B. 30s
C. 40s
D. 50s
E. 60s

56. Which **single** type of malignant thyroid cancer is the most common?

A. Anaplastic
B. Follicular
C. Hürthle cell
D. Lymphoma
E. Papillary

57. Risk factors for breast cancer include all of the following **except**:

A. Breastfeeding
B. Early menarche
C. First pregnancy > 30 years old
D. Late menopause
E. Nulliparity

58–61. ECG abnormalities

A. 1st degree heart block
B. 2nd degree heart block (Mobitz type I–Wenckebach phenomenon)
C. 2nd degree heart block (Mobitz type II)
D. 3rd degree heart block
E. Left bundle branch block
F. Right bundle branch block
G. Wolff–Parkinson–White syndrome

For each of the ECG findings below select the **single** most appropriate diagnosis from the above list.

58. The initial PR interval is normal but progressively lengthens with each successive beat until AV transmission is blocked completely and the P-wave is not followed by a QRS complex. The cycle then repeats itself.

59. The PR interval is uniformly prolonged in each cycle. All P waves are followed by a QRS complex and the PR interval remains constant.

60. The QRS is > 0.12 s with inverted T-waves in leads I, AVL and V5-6.

61. The PR interval is constant, normal or prolonged, but not all P-waves are followed by a QRS complex.

62. The NSF for Diabetes has suggested that the ideal target HbA1C should be less than or equal to:

   A. 5.4%
   B. 6.0%
   C. 6.5%
   D. 7.0%
   E. 7.4%

63–66. Oral hypoglycaemics

   A. Alpha-glucosidase inhibitor
   B. Biguanide
   C. Glitazones
   D. Post-prandial glucose regulators
   E. Sulphonylureas

Match the class of oral hypoglycaemic agents with their correct primary mode of action. Each option may be used once, more than once or not at all.

63. Decreases hepatic glucose production.

64. Stimulates insulin secretion by β-cells (**two** answers).

65. Delays absorption of carbohydrate.

66. Decreases insulin resistance and resensitizes the body to its own insulin.

67. Which **two** statements are correct regarding treatment of vulvo-vaginal candidiasis, based on evidence?

   A. Nystatin pessaries should be inserted at night for at least 7 days.
   B. Oral fluconazole may be prescribed as a single dose of 150 mg.
   C. Oral itraconazole has been associated with reports of heart failure.
   D. Oral ketaconazole requires baseline serum liver function tests.
   E. Treating a woman's male sexual partner significantly improves resolution of the woman's symptoms and reduces the rate of symptomatic relapse.

68–73. Antithrombotic therapy in peripheral vascular disease

    A. Aspirin or clopidogrel
    B. Consider aspirin plus dipyridamole
    C. Consider warfarin
    D. Heparin and angioplasty
    E. Intra-arterial thrombolysis or early surgery
    F. Intravenous heparin and emergency surgery intervention

For each of the clinical conditions below select the **single** most appropriate form of antithrombotic therapy from the above list. Each option may be used once, more than once or not at all.

68. Carotid endarterectomy

69. Symptomatic carotid stenosis but unfit for surgery (**two** possible answers)

70. Embolic arterial occlusion

71. Intermittent claudication

72. Diabetes

73. Acute or chronic arterial occlusion (**two** possible answers)

74. Which of the following is **not** a test for female infertility:

    A. Serum FSH taken between days 2 and 5 of the menstrual cycle
    B. Serum LH taken 5–10 days before menstruation
    C. Serum progesterone taken 5–10 days prior to menstruation
    D. Serum prolactin
    E. Serum TSH

75. First-line drug treatment for patients with heart failure due to left ventricular systolic dysfunction should be (unless contraindicated):

    A. ACE inhibitor
    B. Angiotensin II-receptor antagonist
    C. Beta-blocker
    D. Diuretic
    E. Spironolactone

76. Maximum predicted heart rate is calculated as _____ minus half the patient's age for men:

A. 205
B. 210
C. 220
D. 230
E. 240

77. The following are components of *Good Medical Practice* except:

A. If you have grounds to believe that a doctor is putting patients at risk, you must inform the primary care trust.
B. In an emergency, wherever it may arise, you must offer anyone at risk the assistance you could reasonably be expected to provide.
C. You may end a relationship with a patient solely on the basis of a complaint about you.
D. You should offer an apology, when appropriate, if a patient under your care has suffered harm.
E. You should inform the patient, orally or in writing, why you have decided to end the professional relationship.

78. According to the Royal College of Obstetrics and Gynaecology and GMC, chaperones should be offered for which of the following cases:

A. A female doctor examining a female patient's breasts
B. A female doctor performing a PV exam in a female patient
C. A female doctor performing a PR exam on a male patient
D. A male doctor performing a PV exam in a female patient
E. A male doctor performing a PR exam on a male patient

79. A 40-year-old woman presents to your evening surgery with an acute exacerbation of asthma. Her usual peak flow is 390 LPM. Her predicted peak flow is 440 LPM. Her peak flow now is 200 LPM. Her current inhalers are salbutamol and seretide 500. The RR is 20 and pulse 96. On chest examination there are bilateral wheezes and tightness. She has audible wheezes and is SOB at rest. The **single** most appropriate treatment is:

A. Call 999 for a blue light ambulance
B. Prescribe a 7-day course of 30 mg of prednisolone od
C. Prescribe a volumatic spacer and instruct her to put 12 puffs of salbutamol into the spacer and inhale
D. Prescribe a week's course of amoxycillin and prednisolone
E. Start nebulizer treatment with salbutamol and ipratropium

80. A 45-year-old patient with type 2 diabetes on metformin continues to have a HbA1C of 9 for 6 months despite drug compliance. His BMI is 30. According to evidence-based medicine, the **single** most appropriate step is to:

A. Add acarbose
B. Add glitazone
C. Change to sulfonylurea
D. Convert to insulin therapy
E. Offer sibutramine

81. A 13-year-old girl presents with mild acne vulgaris. The **single** most appropriate treatment is:

A. Benzoyl peroxide
B. Dianette
C. Isotretinoin
D. Oral doxycycline
E. Oxytetracycline

82. The following statements regarding acute cholecystitis are correct **except:**

A. Delayed or 'interval' surgery is preferable to early cholecystectomy.
B. First-line treatment includes nil by mouth, IV fluids and analgesia.
C. It is most often caused by gallstones.
D. Patients suspected of having acute cholecystitis should be referred to hospital immediately.
E. Percutaneous cholecystostomy is a safe alternative to cholecystectomy for those unfit for a GA.

83. The following statements regarding the NICE guidance on the treatment of generalized anxiety disorder (Dec 2004) are correct **except:**

A. Benzodiazepines have been implicated in up to 10% of road traffic accidents.
B. Buspirone Improves symptoms in the long term.
C. Cognitive therapy focuses on patients' current problems and not their past.
D. The best treatment of all is cognitive therapy.
E. There is no significant difference between paroxetine and venlafaxine in reducing symptoms in the short term.

84. Presentations for head and neck cancer include all of the following **except:**

   A. Cervicalgia
   B. Cervical lymph node enlargement
   C. Dysphagia
   D. Earache
   E. Hoarseness

85–90. Headaches

   A. Cluster
   B. Idiopathic intracranial hypertension
   C. Intracranial tumour
   D. Medication overuse
   E. Meningitis
   F. Migraine
   G. Primary angle closure glaucoma
   H. Subacute carbon monoxide poisoning
   I. Subarachnoid haemorrhage
   J. Temporal arteritis
   K. Tension

For each of the patients below select the **single** most likely diagnosis from the above list of options:

85. A 45-year-old bus driver reports a tightness around his head, spreading into the neck. It lasts a few hours at a time.

86. A 20-year-old heavy smoker reports spells of headaches lasting 2–3 months each year. He has pain around his left eye, mostly at night. He has to bang his head against the wall, as the pain is intolerable. The pain lasts for an hour. On examination the eye is red and watering with blocked nose.

87. A 55-year-old woman reports persistent headache, worse at night. On examination there is marked scalp tenderness.

88. A 50-year-old woman reports headache, nausea, mild eye pain and sees coloured haloes around lights.

89. A 25-year-old woman reports headaches, nausea, vomiting, giddiness, dimness and double vision. She and her husband are renovating an old property.

90. A 50-year-old man complains of severe headache and neck stiffness after a stag night. It is now the worst he has ever had.

91. Which **three** of the following are cardinal signs of glaucoma?

A. Increased intraocular pressure
B. Optic disc cupping
C. Proptosis
D. Squint
E. Visual field constriction

92. Which **single** best treatment is advised for acute cluster headache?

A. Analgesia
B. Ergotamine
C. Lithium carbonate
D. Methysergide
E. Sumatriptan

93. Which **three** drugs may be used to treat menstrually related migraines?

A. Amitriptyline
B. Beta-blockers
C. Continuous combined oral contraceptives for 9 weeks
D. Mefenamic acid
E. Transdermal oestrogen patches twice weekly

94. The **single** non-invasive investigation of choice for the diagnosis of clinically suspected deep venous thrombosis is:

A. Compression ultrasonography
B. Fibrin D-dimer
C. Impedance plethysmography
D. Magnetic resonance venography
E. Spiral computed tomography

95. The **single** preferred imaging method to distinguish Parkinson's disease from essential tremor is:

A. CT scan
B. FP-CIT (DaTSCAN)
C. Magnetoencephalography
D. MRI scan
E. MR spectroscopy

96. High 'pathological' myopia is a risk factor for all of the following eye conditions **except**:

A. Central retinal vein occlusion
B. Glaucoma
C. Macular degeneration
D. Retinal detachment
E. Strabismus

97. Select **two** correct statements regarding head lice:

A. Bedding must be boiled at a temperature above 60°C
B. Treatment with lotion requires two 2-hour treatments 1 week apart.
C. Infestation is heaviest behind the ears and in the occipital region
D. They are transmitted by hopping.
E. Treatment with malathion is more effective than wet-combing.

98–101. Leg swelling

A. Cellulitis
B. Chronic lymphoedema
C. Congestive heart failure
D. Deep vein thrombosis
E. Ruptured Baker's cyst

For each of the clinical cases below select the **single** most likely diagnosis from the above list of options:

98. A 66-year-old woman complains of swelling of the entire length of the left leg. On examination, the circumference of the left leg is 4 cm greater than that of the right leg with pitting ankle oedema. She also complains of pain and has moderate varicose veins. She has a history of atrial fibrillation and hypertension.

99. A 60-year-old obese woman presents with non-pitting oedema in both lower legs following bilateral knee replacement.

100. A 65-year-old woman presents with SOB at rest and gross dependent oedema in both legs with breakdown of overlying skin. On examination she has an enlarged tender liver and basal crepitations.

101. A 70-year-old woman with generalized osteoarthritis presents with stiffness and swelling of the right lower leg and popliteal fossa of the knee.

102. Bulimia may be associated with all of the following **except**:

    A. Binge drinking
    B. Bipolar disorder
    C. Normal weight
    D. Score lines on the backs of the hands (Russell's sign)
    E. Swollen parotid glands

103. The **single** initial investigation to exclude left ventricular heart failure is:

    A. Brain natriuretic peptide
    B. Cardiac enzymes
    C. Chest x-ray
    D. Echocardiogram
    E. 12-lead ECG

104. A 60-year-old woman presents with bruising. She has a history of gout. On examination, the spleen is enlarged. The white cell and platelet counts are both elevated, and there is an increase in red blood cell mass. The **single** most likely diagnosis is:

    A. Acute leukaemia
    B. Essential thrombocythaemia
    C. Multiple myeloma
    D. Polycythaemia rubra vera
    E. Primary myelosclerosis

105. The **single** best treatment for this woman is:

    A. Busulfan
    B. Hydroxyurea
    C. Melphalan
    D. Supportive
    E. Venesection

106. A 40-year-old man complains of shoulder pain. On examination he has pain when abducting his shoulder 45 degrees above and below the horizontal. Pain is also elicited on pushing down on his raised arm. The **single** most likely diagnosis is:

    A. Adhesive capsulitis
    B. Cervical spondylosis
    C. Glenohumeral subluxation
    D. Injury of the spinal accessory nerve
    E. Rotator cuff tendinitis

107. Psoriasis may be exacerbated by all of the following factors **except:**

A. Alcohol
B. Beta-blockers
C. NSAIDs
D. Sunlight
E. Tonsillitis treated with antibiotics

108–112. Treatment for conditions of the nails

A. Dovonex scalp application to nails
B. Gentamicin ear drops
C. Gloves and moisturizer
D. Lamisil
E. Sporanox
F. Topical steroid

For each of the conditions below, select the **single** most effective treatment from the above list:

108. Lamellar splitting

109. *Candida* paronychia

110. Pseudomonal nail infection

111. Psoriasis nails

112. Irritant hand eczema

113–120. Treatment for dermatological conditions

A. Duoderm
B. Efudix (topical 5-FU)
C. Epiderm + Cocois
D. Intradermal triamcinolone
E. Iontophoresis
F. Mepiform
G. Mepitel
H. Prednisolone
I. PUVA

For each of the dermatological conditions listed below select the **single** most effective treatment from the above list of options:

113. Palmar hyperhydrosis

114. Granuloma annulare

115. Keloid

116. Bowen's disease on the lower leg

117. Actinic keratosis

118. Pityriasis capitis

119. Venous ulcer

120. Bullous pemphigoid

121–127. Statistics

    A. Absolute risk
    B. Attributable risk
    C. Mean
    D. Median
    E. Mode
    F. Negative predictive value
    G. Numbers needed to treat
    H. Odds ratio
    I. Positive predictive value
    J. Relative risk
    K. Sensitivity
    L. Specificity

Match each of the definitions below with the correct term above:

121. The most common value observed.

122. The proportion of patients with a positive test correctly identified as having the disease.

123. The proportion of true negatives correctly identified by the test.

124. Incidence of disease in the exposed population divided by the incidence of disease in the non-exposed population.

125. Incidence of disease in the exposed population minus the incidence of disease in the non-exposed population.

126. The inverse of (% treated group with the desired outcome minus % controls with the desired outcome), i.e. 1/ARR%.

127. If pill users are at 2 × more risk of a DVT than non-pill users, this value is 2. It is equal to (the number of pill users with DVT multiplied by the number of non-pill users with no DVT) divided by (the number of non-pill users with DVT multiplied by the number of pill-users without DVT).

128, 129. If 40 out of 200 heroin misusers in the treated subutex group give up heroin and 4 out of 200 give up heroin in the control group, then:

A. 5
B. 6
C. 10
D. 18
E. 36

128. The absolute risk reduction % is?

129. The NNT is?

130. Select **two** cardinal signs of retinal detachment:

A. Coloured haloes
B. Curtain falling over vision
C. Flashing lights
D. Painful loss of vision
E. Red eye

131. Select **two** correct statements regarding central retinal vein occlusion:

A. The fundus appears like a stormy red sea.
B. It causes painful loss of vision.
C. It is less common than arterial occlusion.
D. There is no definitive treatment.
E. Visual acuity may be reduced to finger counting.

132. Select **two** cardinal signs of diabetic retinopathy:

    A. Arteriovenous nipping
    B. Copper-wiring of arteries
    C. Grey opalescent retina
    D. Microaneurysms
    E. Yellow hard exudates

133. Indications for colposcopy referral include all of the following **except**:

    A. HPV testing
    B. 2nd occurrence of mild dyskaryosis
    C. 3 consecutive inadequate smears
    D. Moderate dyskaryosis
    E. Suspicious-looking cervix

134. The following statements regarding the Mental Health NSF are correct **except**:

    A. 1:6 patients have mental health problems.
    B. 1:250 patients have bipolar affective disorder or schizophrenia.
    C. 90% of carers who live with a person with a serious mental illness suffer from depression.
    D. Performance is assessed by the National Psychiatric Morbidity Survey.
    E. Standard 3 makes it mandatory to provide 24-hour Section 12-approved doctor and ASW care.

135–137. Management of mental illness

    A. Continue antidepressant for 2 more weeks
    B. Increase the dose of antidepressant or consider switching to another
    C. Prescribe antipsychotic
    D. Prescribe antidepressant
    E. Refer to psychiatric outpatient clinic
    F. Urgent referral for sectioning

For each of the patients below select the **single** most appropriate management from the above list of options:

135. The mother of a 20-year-old unemployed man is concerned, since her son has not left his room for 3 months. The son agrees for you to visit him at home and during your visit you find him aloof. You determine that he does not have psychotic features.

136. You are contacted by the neighbour of a 25-year-old woman. You contact the woman, who agrees for you to visit her at home. Upon arrival you see that there is broken window glass, used syringes, beer bottles scattered on the floor. She reports that she cannot sleep as she hears shouting voices in her head.

137. A 35-year-old man on Prozac states that nothing has happened in 4 weeks. He asks whether he can try a different antidepressant.

138. Which **five** of the following blood tests should be arranged for a patient suspected of having Alzheimer's disease?

   A. B_{12} and folate
   B. Bone profile
   C. Fasting lipids
   D. FBC + ESR
   E. Hepatitis virology
   F. HIV
   G. U+E + glucose
   H. LFTs
   I. Syphilis serology
   J. TFTs

139. Drug levels are required for all of the following medications **except**:

   A. Carbamazepine
   B. Ciclosporin
   C. Digoxin
   D. Lithium
   E. Theophylline

140. The following statements are correct regarding severe acute respiratory syndrome (SARS) **except**:

   A. Chest x-ray shows changes suggestive of pneumonia.
   B. Early antibiotic intervention is effective.
   C. The incubation period is between 2 and 7 days.
   D. There have been documented mortalities in Hong Kong and Vietnam.
   E. 20 ml of blood in a plain glass tube should be taken.

141. The **single** gold standard for detecting the hepatitis C viral RNA genome is:

   A. Elevated alanine aminotransferase
   B. ELISA-3 blood test
   C. Liver biopsy
   D. Polymerase chain reaction (PCR)

142. The following statements regarding fitness to drive are correct except:

A. A diabetic patient is required to notify the DVLA if on tablets.
B. An HGV driver who has suffered an MI is permanently banned from driving.
C. A licence may be granted for up to 3 years if a patient has been seizure-free for 1 year.
D. A patient may be granted a licence to drive if he/she has only had seizures during sleep for the past 3 years.
E. A patient with 6/10 corrected vision is not banned from driving.

143–147. PV bleed

A. Inevitable abortion
B. Missed abortion
C. Placenta abruptio
D. Placenta praevia
E. Threatened abortion

For each of the patients below select the **single** most likely diagnosis from the above list of options:

143. A 6/40 pregnant female presents with PV spotting. On PV exam the os is closed.

144. A 8/40 pregnant female presents with PV bleeding. On PV exam the os is open.

145. A 14/40 pregnant female is noted to have a uterus that is small for dates. The os is closed.

146. A 22/40 pregnant female comes for an antenatal check. No fetal heart sounds are present.

147. A 29/40 pregnant female presents with severe lower abdominal pain and PV bleed.

148–150. Methotrexate

A. Continue current dose of methotrexate
B. Decrease by 2.5 mg weekly
C. Discontinue methotrexate
D. Increase by 2.5 mg weekly

A patient has been recently started on methotrexate for rheumatoid arthritis. He has regular FBC tests. For each of the results below, select the **single** most appropriate management plan from the above list of options:

148. The WCC was 8×10^9/L and platelets 220×10^9/L in October and 2 months later the WCC is now 3×10^9/L and the platelets 100×10^9/L.

149. The patient complains of a cough. On examination he is afebrile and the chest is clear. The WCC is 11×10^9/L and the platelets are 200×10^9/L.

150. The patient reports symptoms only mildly improving on methotrexate. She is still in considerable pain. The WCC is 12×10^9/L and the platelet count is 250×10^9/L.

151. Causes of monocular diplopia include all of the following **except**:

A. Astigmatism
B. Cataract
C. Dislocated lens
D. Pterygium
E. Strabismus

152. Bisphosphonates are indicated for all of the following conditions **except**:

A. Inflammatory bowel conditions requiring oral corticosteroids
B. Postmenopausal Muslim women
C. Postmenopausal osteoporosis
D. Premenopausal women with a family history of osteoporosis
E. Prolonged oral corticosteroid use for more than 3 months

153. A 14-year-old boy has persistent otitis externa. He enjoys swimming. He has been using Otomise spray. The ear swab result is positive for *Pseudomonas aeruginosa*. The **single** best management option is:

    A. Add amoxicillin
    B. Add ciprofloxacin
    C. Add trimethoprim
    D. Advise him to continue to use the Otomise spray
    E. Advise him to wear ear plugs when swimming

154. A 20-year-old professional rugby player develops infectious mononucleosis. He wants to know if and when he will be fit to go back to contact sports. The **single** best management option is:

    A. Advise to wait 6 weeks
    B. Advise to wait 3 months
    C. Advise to return when monospot test is negative
    D. Arrange for a CT scan of the liver and spleen
    E. Arrange for an ultrasound of the spleen to exclude splenomegaly

155. The following are appropriate diagnostic investigations for fever following tropical travel **except**:

    A. CRP
    B. 3 EDTA samples to haematology for thick and thin films
    C. Malaria serology
    D. Stool for parasites and culture with mention of countries visited
    E. Tropical serology for schistosomiasis

156–162. Statistics

    A. Absolute
    B. Attributable
    C. Case-referent
    D. Cohort
    E. Cross-sectional
    F. Incidence
    G. Odds
    H. Prevalence
    I. Relative

    For each of the numbered gaps, choose one **single** word from the above list that best completes the sentence. Each word may be used once, more than once, or not at all.

    (156) _____ rate is defined as the number of new cases in a given period divided by the total person time at risk during the period. (157) _____ratio is good to study large populations and rare diseases. (158) _____study looks back from disease to exposure. It gives a comparison of (159) _____ rates. (160) _____ study looks forward from exposure to disease. Both (161) ____ risk and (162) _____ ratio can be determined with this study. However, this study is time-consuming.

163. A 10-year-old girl presents with persistent productive cough for 4 months with no relief from repeated courses of antibiotics. On chest examination she has occasional wheezes. Which **two** investigations should be arranged?

A. Chest x-ray
B. Refer to paediatric outpatient clinic
C. Sweat test
D. Urgent referral to chest clinic for Tb testing
E. Ventolin challenge (4 puffs through spacer) and check lung function test

164. Prophylactic antibiotics should be prescribed in HIV-positive patients, if the CD4 count drops below:

A. 100 cells/mm^3
B. 200 cells/mm^3
C. 300 cells/mm^3
D. 400 cells/mm^3
E. 500 cells/mm^3

165–168. ECG arrhythmias

A. Atrial fibrillation
B. Atrial flutter
C. Atrial tachycardia
D. Sinus tachycardia
E. Ventricular tachycardia
F. Ventricular fibrillation
G. Wolff–Parkinson–White syndrome

For each of the numbered gaps, choose one **single** option from the above list that best completes the sentence. Each word may be used once, more than once, or not at all.

In (165) _____, the P-waves are absent. The atrial rate is between 350 and 600 beats/min and the ventricular rate is between 100 and 180 beats/min. In (166) _____ the atrial impulses can be conducted via the accessory pathway, causing ventricular pre-excitation and broad QRS complexes with delta waves. This accessory pathway allows for very fast ventricular rates, which puts the patient at risk of (167) _____. (168) _____ is defined as 3 or more ventricular extrasystoles in succession at a rate of more than 120 beats/min. The QRS complexes are monomorphic or polymorphic.

169. A 56-year-old obese man presents with sudden onset of severe back pain. He has no signs of sciatica or urinary incontinence. BP is 150/90. Possible diagnoses include all of the following **except**:

A. Acute pancreatitis
B. Cord compression
C. Renal colic
D. Ruptured abdominal aortic aneurysm
E. Simple mechanical back pain

170. According to evidence-based medicine, which of the following OTC cough medicines are recommended for acute cough in adults:

A. Antihistamines
B. Antitussives
C. Expectorants
D. Mucolytics
E. None of the above

171–176. Treatment of dermatological conditions

A. Aciclovir
B. Betnovate + Diprobase + Atarax nocte
C. Capasal shampoo
D. Diprosalic ointment until better + hydrocortisone cream to other areas
E. Elocon
F. Erythroped, Differin + Dianette (triple therapy)
G. Fusidin H
H. Lamisil (terbinafine) crushed tablet od for 1 month
I. Occlusal paint
J. Refer for Roaccutane

For each of the patients below select the **single** most appropriate treatment from the above list of options. Each option may be used once, more than once or not at all.

171. A 2-year-old boy presents with eczema over his elbows and thighs.

172. A 3-year-old boy presents with a wart on his scalp.

173. A 2-year-old girl presents with eczema herpeticum over the face and body: (Select **two** best answers)

174. A 6-year-old girl presents with eczema over the back of her elbows, popliteal fossa, and her lower back.

175. A 14-year-old girl presents with severe acne over her face, arms and back. She has tried topical therapy without success.

176. A 4-year-old Afro-Caribbean boy presents with scalp ringworm, hair loss and posterior cervical lymphadenopathy.

177–183. Algorithm for treatment of breast cancer

- A. Axillary node clearance
- B. Axillary node sampling
- C. ± chemo
- D. Chemotherapy
- E. DXT
- F. ± tamoxifen
- G. Tamoxifen
- H. Wide local excision
- I. ± Zoladex

For each of the numbered gaps, choose a **single** management option from the above list that best completes the algorithm. Each option may be used once, more than once or not at all.

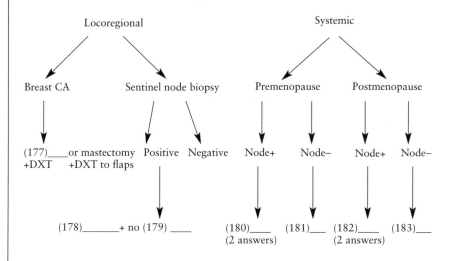

184. An 80-year-old woman requests a laxative for constipation secondary to codeine-containing analgesia. The following are suitable management options **except**:

A. Change analgesia
B. Prescribe co-danthromer
C. Prescribe lactulose
D. Prescribe senna
E. Suggest increase fruit and bran in diet

185. According to the NICE Cancer Referral Guidelines for Suspected Cancer (June 2005), the following clinical features warrant urgent referral to breast clinic **except**:

A. A 22-year-old woman presents with bilateral painful breasts.
B. A 30-year-old woman presents with a discrete mass persisting after next period.
C. A 20-year-old woman presents with spontaneous right-sided blood-stained nipple. She has no family history of breast cancer.
D. A 35-year-old woman has persistent right nipple eczema unresponsive to treatment.
E. A 50-year-old man with a left-sided firm, subareolar mass.

186. The following statements regarding buprenorphine (Subutex) are correct **except**:

A. It can only be prescribed by GPs with a specialist interest in drug misuse.
B. It is a Class C drug according to the Misuse of Drugs Act 1971.
C. It may be used as substitution therapy for patients with moderate opioid dependence.
D. Patients on methadone should be down to 30 mg of methadone od prior to conversion to Subutex.
E. Should be taken at least 4 hours after last use of opioid.

187. The following statements regarding the NICE guidelines on Alzheimer's are correct **except**:

A. Drug treatment may continue solely on the basis of improvement in the MMSE score.
B. GPs should not initiate therapy with acetylcholinesterase-inhibiting drugs.
C. MMSE score should be above 12 to consider treatment with donepezil.
D. Patients should be reassessed every 6 months.
E. The patient should be reassessed 2–4 months after the maintenance dose has been established.

188. The following are risk factors for a patient's risk of danger to others **except:** (Source: Dual diagnosis team SLAM)

A. Evidence of general self-neglect
B. Lack of remorse regarding re violence
C. Morbid jealousy
D. Past history of violence with alcohol or drugs
E. Persisting denial of responsibility

189–192. Hepatitis B serology results

A. Immune, post-vaccination
B. Immune, past exposure to HBV
C. Infected, low risk of transmission
D. Infected, high risk of transmission

For each of the HBV serology results listed below select the **single** most appropriate interpretation from the above list of options:

189. sAb +ve   sAg –ve   cAb –ve   eAg –ve   eAb –ve   DNA –ve

190. sAb –ve   sAg +ve   cAb +ve   eAg +ve   eAb –ve   DNA +ve

191. sAb –ve   sAg +ve   cAb +ve   eAg –ve   eAb +ve   DNA –ve

192. sAb +ve   sAg –ve   cAb +ve   eAg –ve   eAb +ve   DNA –ve

193. Which **one** of the following statements is incorrect regarding ischaemic events:

A. Age is the main risk factor for a stroke.
B. Anticoagulation is offered routinely for stroke patients.
C. Carotid stenosis of > 70% is an indication for endarterectomy.
D. Overall thrombolytic therapy is associated with a significant increase in death from haemorrhage within 7–10 days.
E. The ESPRIT study showed that aspirin + dipyridamole were better than aspirin alone following ischaemic events.

194. What is the second-line drug treatment for bipolar disorder?

A. Carbamazepine
B. Fluoxetine
C. Lithium
D. Valproate
E. Venlafaxine

195. The following conditions may be associated with alopecia **except:**

    A. Chronic iron deficiency
    B. Fungal scalp infection
    C. Hyperthyroidism
    D. Polycystic ovarian syndrome
    E. Warfarin

196–200. Contraception

    A. Arrange for urgent IUCD insertion
    B. Prescribe Levonelle-2
    C. Suggest Depo-Provera IM
    D. Suggest Mirena coil
    E. Switch to Brevinor
    F. Switch to Eugynon
    G. Switch to Femodette
    H. Switch to Micronor
    I. Use condoms for 1 week

196. A 25-year-old woman complains of breakthrough bleeding on Microgynon 30. Her smear test, swabs and speculum exam are all normal.

197. A 17-year-old girl has had UPSI 4 days prior and seeks contraception.

198. A 35-year-old woman complains of breakthrough bleeding on Micronor. She smokes 20 cigarettes a day and has lactose intolerance. Her smear test, swabs and speculum exam are all normal.

199. A 19-year-old girl has recently had a TOP. She reports that she is too forgetful to remember to take pills every day.

200. A 40-year-old woman forgot to take her Micronor pill yesterday. She comes to you for advice. You suggest she take yesterday's and today's pill and advise that she....?

Applied Knowledge Test Module Paper Three: Answers

1. D

2. H

3. A

4. E

5. F

6. C

7. F

8. G

9. A

10. I

11. E

12. N

13. C or B

14. B or C

15. F or H

16. H or F

17. O

18. I

19. J.   Responsibility for OOHs is to be assumed by the PCO. OOHs includes 6:30 p.m. to 8.00 a.m., weekends and bank holidays and would cost GPs £6000 or 7% of the global sum calculation.

20. L

21. F

22. H

23. P.   This is approximately 20–25% less than actual list size and is based on a formula that incorporates age, gender, list turnover, morbidity and mortality, nursing home/residential home consults, rurality and market forces.

24. E.   London boroughs such as Hackney or Tower Hamlets are worse hit. Basic knowledge of the principles behind the new contract is also important for the viva. The alternative would be to remain in a PMS practice or go private.

25. D.   According to the RCGP guidelines reinforced by the Faculty of Occupational Medicine, bedrest is no longer advocated. The patient should resume normal activities with adequate analgesia for simple mechanical backache.

26. B.   This patient has a series of red flag signs (age of onset over 55, structural abnormality, weight loss and widespread neurological signs). Other red flags include non-mechanical pain, presentation under age 20, and past history of carcinoma, HIV or steroids.

27. F.   This patient has nerve root pain, which should resolve with conservative management.

28. E.   This patient has signs of a cauda equina syndrome (gait disturbance, saddle anaesthesia and sphincter disturbance) requiring urgent decompression.

29. C. This man may have psychosocial 'yellow flags' such as a belief that the back pain is harmful or potentially severely disabling, a fear-avoidance behaviour and reduced activity levels, tendency to low mood and withdrawal from social interaction or expectation of passive treatment(s) rather than a belief that active participation will help. Yellow flags are associated with poor outcomes. Referral for reactivation/rehabilitation should be considered in patients who fail to return to work by 6 weeks.

30. D

31. E

32. H

33. A

34. G

35. B

36. F

37. E. Tympanosclerosis is an incidental finding and may be associated with past scarring of the TM. No treatment is necessary. Do not try to remove this 'cotton wool' appearance to the drum mistaking it as a foreign body, lest you perforate the eardrum! I have seen this happen in A&E.

38. ABC. Also, if you have been taking this medicine for more than 3 weeks, the dose should be reduced gradually when you stop taking steroids unless your doctor says otherwise.

39. B

40. D. If you do not put the female symbol or at least write 'for coc' on the prescription, the patient will not be charged NHS prescription costs but instead private prescription charges. Without the symbol, the prescription indicates a private prescription for use for acne and not an NHS prescription for contraception.

41. AH

42. AH.   If the patient has missed methadone for 3 days, he will need to be restarted on methadone at much lower doses and not his current dose, so he should not be offered a repeat prescription.

43. F.   This man has a dual diagnosis – mental illness and drug misuse.

44. G.   Antabuse is reserved for mantaining patients off-alcohol following an inpatient detoxification.

45. B.   Some may advocate maintaining a patient on diazepam with a history of long-term use, but in the long run slow weaning is more advisable.

46. C

47. DE

48. C

49. B.   Leflunomide is a new DMD (disease-modifying drug) for the treatment of rheumatoid arthritis. It is very popular in the US and is now available on NHS prescription. Patient's BP and serum LFTs should be monitored.

50. D.   Treatment is symptomatic, with foot rest or wearing a walking plaster.

51. H.   Classic symptoms for plantar fasciitis which may be treated with NSAIDs or steroid injection.

52. J.   Radionuclide bone scans will show this March fracture.

53. F.   Pain occurs from pressure on an interdigital neuroma, which may require excision.

54. B. Osteochondritis dissecans or Freiberg's infarction presents with forefoot pain around puberty, especially in girls. Treatment involves good shoes ± metatarsal pad and limited activity for 4–6 weeks.

55. BC

56. E

57. A

58. B

59. A

60. C

61. E

62. E

63. B

64. DE

65. A

66. C

67. BC. Treatment with nystatin requires at least 14 days!

68. A

69. B or C

70. F

71. A

72. A

73. D or E

74. B.   The FSH and LH tests should be performed in the early follicular phase. If > 10 IU/L, the patient should receive an early referral.

75. A.   First-line treatment should be an ACE inhibitor. The second-line drug is ARB. Then add in a beta-blocker. For NYHA III or IV, spironolactone is recommended but beware of deteriorating renal function.

76. A.   For women it is 220 minus the patient's age. Hard exercise pushes the heart to 70–89% of MHR. Moderate exercise is 50–69% of MHR and light exercise is 30–49% of MHR. Before signing someone fit for exercise, ensure they do not have any coronary heart disease risk factors. If this is the case, a specialist opinion is mandatory and you may not certify the patient fit for the gym or exercise. Exercise on prescription may be used to treat mild to moderate depression (three times weekly) and to treat obesity (five times weekly).

77. C.   Obtain a copy of *Good Medical Practice* from the GMC.

78. ABCDE.   In July 2002, the RCOG published *Gynaecological Examinations: Guidelines for Specialist Practice*, which incorporates the guidelines of the GMC's Standards Committee and covers use of chaperones.

79. E.   If her peak flow does not improve, call 999.

80. B.   According to 'Treating to Target' guidance launched at the Diabetes UK Conference in 2003, a step-up treatment is advised if the HbA1C is persistently > 7.

81. A.   Topical treatment is suggested for at least 3 months. Alternative topical treatment is Zineryt (erythromycin and zinc).

82. A.   Vice versa is true.

83. B. Buspirone may improve symptoms in the short term.

84. A. Squamous cell CA of the head and neck constitutes 5% of all the cancers in the UK. People in their 40s and 50s are most at risk. Risk factors include alcohol, smoking and having a poor diet.

85. K

86. A

87. J

88. G

89. H

90. I

91. ABE

92. E. The rest are examples of prophylactic treatment except for analgesia, which plays no role in the treatment of cluster headaches.

93. CDE

94. A

95. B

96. A

97. CE. Treatment requires 12 hours or overnight treatment once weekly × 2.

98. D

99. B

100. C

101. E

102. B

103. A

104. D

105. E. Hydroxyurea is then prescribed if the platelet count or white cell count is difficult to control.

106. E. The painful arc sign is elicited between 60 and 120 degrees of abduction.

107. D. Sunlight exposure improves psoriasis.

108. C. Lamellar splitting results from detergents, trauma or water.

109. E. Sporanox (itraconazole) is prescribed as 200 mg bd 7/7 repeated monthly for 2 pulses.

110. B

111. A. This subungual or periungual topical therapy is applied for 2 months. Elocon lotion is an alternative.

112. F

113. E

114. I

115. F.   This silicon dressing is now available on NHS prescription and costs £30 for 10 dressings.

116. B.   Excision and grafting is an alternative treatment.

117. B.   Other treatment options include cryotherapy, Solease 3% (topical diclofenac), surgery or photodynamic therapy.

118. C.   Epiderm is a soap substitute and should be applied overnight to the scalp and washed out to descale the scalp. Then Cocois should be applied at half-inch intervals.

119. G.   Mepitel is a non-adherent silicone dressing used for leg ulcers, decubitus ulcers and burns.

120. H.   Azathioprine may also be added.

121. E

122. I

123. L

124. J

125. B

126. G.   NNT, absolute risk and relative risk have all appeared in previous exams. You must know how to calculate these values given an example.

127. H

128. D.   20% − 2% = 18%

129. B   1/18% = 5.56 or 6 people

130. BC. It causes painless loss of vision and is an ophthalmological emergency.

131. AE

132. DE. Degrees of diabetic retinopathy increase in severity from BDR (background retinopathy distinguished by the presence of micro-aneurysms), preproliferative retinopathy (presence of lipoproteins as hard exudates, soft exudates) to proliferative retinopathy with neovascularization. As new vessels are at risk of bleeding, i.e. vitreous haemorrhage or forming scar tissue, and may result in permanent vision loss, diabetic patients should be followed closely with annual specialist eye examinations. Laser treatment is used to get closure of leaky blood vessels or microaneurysms. Panretinal photocoagulation is used to treat neovascularization.

133. A

134. C. The actual value is closer to 50%. As carers are at risk of mental illness, standard 6 is designed to cover this and suggests annual assessment of regular and substantial carers for a person on CPA. Standard 7 takes into account that 50% of suicide is due to mental health problems and ensures that staff members are competent to do a suicide risk assessment. Each of the 7 standards has a designated lead authority.

135. E

136. F

137. A

138. DGHIJ

139. A

140. B. Blood should be taken during the acute and convalescent phase (14 days later) with a 20 mL sample of urine and sent to the local lab marked 'suspected SARS'. A paramyxovirus is suspected at this stage. Cases have occurred in the UK, USA, Canada, Europe and the Far East. There is no cure or prophylactic treatment. SARS is a notifiable disease of exclusion.

141. D.   In October 2003, NICE will be reviewing combination treatment of once-weekly pegylated interferon. Currently the only licensed treatment of hepatitis C is interferon-α. Combination therapy involves oral ribavarin in combination with interferon-α2a or -α2b.

142. B.   He will be banned for 3 months as long as he is symptom-free and passes an exercise stress test.

143. E

144. A

145. B

146. B

147. C

148. C.   Medication errors have occurred with methotrexate. It is a once-weekly drug! Methotrexate must be stopped if any profound drop in WCC or platelets occurs.

149. A

150. D

151. E

152. D.   Once-weekly alendronate (Fosamax) is a convenient form of bis-phosphonate therapy. You are liable as a GP if you fail to prescribe osteoporosis prophylaxis to high-risk patients.

153. B

154. E

155. C. Malaria serology is unhelpful as a diagnostic aid and is very rarely indicated. Initial investigation should always be 3 EDTA tubes for blood film. 1% of cases are now due to HIV seroconversion, which will show atypical lymphocytes on film. Suspect if patient has a rash.

156. F

157. G

158. C

159. F

160. D

161. I

162. G

163. AE. Chest x-ray should be arranged to exclude Tb.

164. B. Patients will be at risk of developing PCP, and Septrin should be prescribed.

165. A

166. G

167. F

168. E

169. B. Beware of sudden onset of severe back pain in men over the age of 55. Do not forget to check the abdomen for a pulsatile AAA.

170. E. Recommendation of OTC cough medicines to patients is not justified by current evidence.

171. D

172. I. Other treatment is liquid nitrogen, which is age dependent, as it may cause some discomfort.

173. AG

174. B. If this does not work, the patient should be referred for TLO1 light cabinet for recalcitrant eczema. Diprobase should be applied while at school and Epaderm for home use. Betnovate can then be changed to Elocon when improving.

175. F. If the patient cannot tolerate erythomycin, trimethoprim may be substiuted. Triple therapy is advised for 4 months. Differin gel should be applied thinly and continued as prophylaxis.

176. H. Lamisil is prescribed according to weight. For instance, a ¼ tablet should be crushed for a child weighing < 20 kg. Treatment is od for 1 month. Apply a toothbrush briskly over the entire scalp and place in a plastic specimen cup for culture. A bacterial swab should also be taken to exclude secondary bacterial infection. To improve pick-up rates, place the swab in the culture medium first, prior to applying to the scalp.

177. H

178. A

179. E

180. DI

181. C. G3 is offered chemo, G2 is offered a chemo trial, and G1 is offered nil.

182. CG

183. F

184. C. Lactulose requires a daily fluid intake of 2 L or else it will cause severe abdominal cramping, and therefore should be avoided in the elderly.

185. A. This patient can be initially managed by the GP.

186. A. Any GP may prescribe buprenorphine, but it is advised that the patient also be involved with a community drug team, who will be able to offer ongoing management advice.

187. A. There has to be improvement in behaviour or function in addition to the MMSE score for continued drug therapy for Alzheimer's.

188. A. This is a risk factor for self-harm.

189. A

190. D

191. C

192. B

193. B. Indications for anti-coagulation include AF, crescendo TIAs with tight carotid stenosis and poor LV function. Patients who have suffered a TIA or stroke should routinely be started on aspirin 300 mg od + 25 mg dipyridamole tds for the first 2 weeks, then changed to aspirin 75 mg od + 200 mg dipyridamole MR bd. If there is a further event, then add clopidogrel 75 mg od.

194. A. Lithium is first-line and carbamazepine second-line. You are often asked for the second-line drug treatment, so be careful when reading the question!

195. C. Hypothyroidism leads to poor hair growth and a coarsening of the hair shaft. The most common cause is fungal scalp infections.

196. F. Eugynon has 100 μg more of levonorgestrel (250 μg) and the same amount of ethinylestradiol (30 μg) as Microgynon.

197. A

198. E. Brevinor is a COC, which contains more norethisterone (500 μg) versus 350 μg in Micronor. It also contains 35 μg of ethinylestradiol. Micronor and Brevinor are non-sugar-coated. Lactose-intolerant individuals should not be offered Microgynon or Microval, which are sugar-coated.

199. C. The IUCD is recommended for emergency contraception for up to 5 days after UPSI.

200. I